AF225963

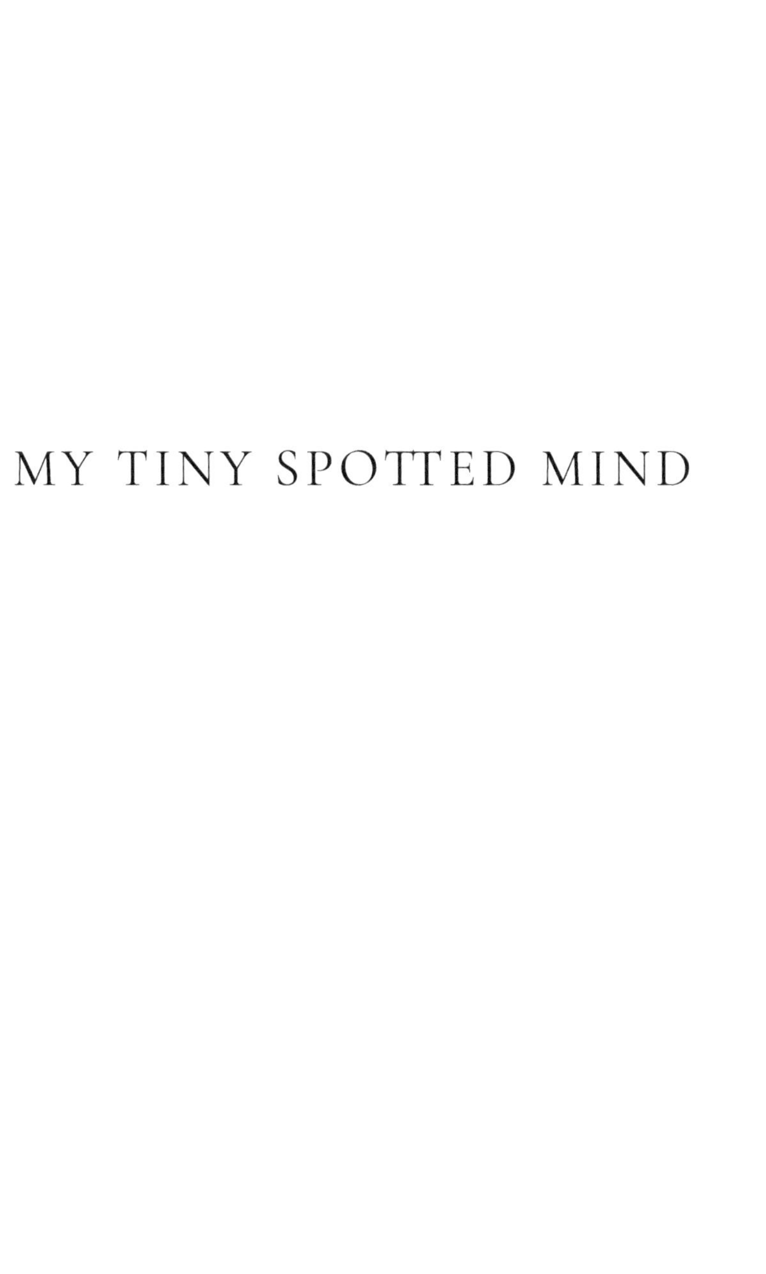

MY TINY SPOTTED MIND

MY TINY SPOTTED MIND

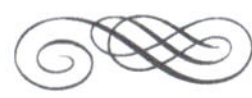

Too Young for MS

DIANA MAISONNEUVE

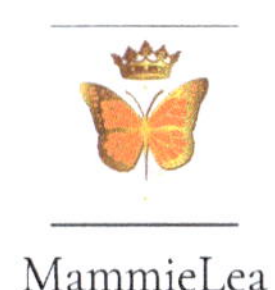

MammieLea

My Tiny Spotted Mind

Too Young for MS

Growing up Black in America with Pediatrics Multiple Sclerosis

First Printing, 2022

Illustration by Haylee Jimeno

Contents

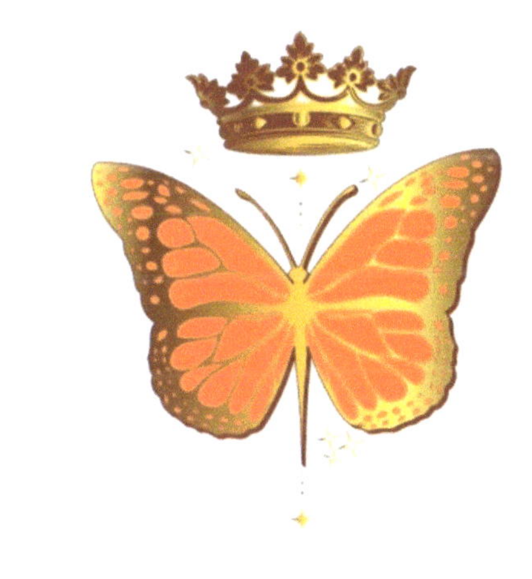

I dedicate this book to honor my two most extraordinary, influential women. My Manmie Lea, your heart has left me so full and taught me that God is love and to love without condition is to be divine. You were the epitome of divinity and possessed the ability to love without reservation and blindly. You framed my faith and intense spirituality, and I know your spirit has guided me through my writing and wellness journey. You were my healer and my internal source of strength. I am also thankful for my incredible mother, who has always been my inspiration, backbone, and anchor. Together these women have taught me a lot about accountability, resiliency, and respect. Through their many life lessons, they kept me grounded. I eventually learned how to harness the ability to balance life with a chronic autoimmune disease. I adopted healthier and more fulfilling practices to appease my pain and understand what God's grace meant.

I worked hard to re-incorporate everything I enjoyed as a child into adulthood without revolving my life around my diagnosis. Through my love of writing, music, exercise, art, perseverance, and obtaining a dream job that allows me to travel the world, I was able to provide myself with wellness. I'm aware that God's mercy engulfs me because of obstacles I couldn't bare alone as an adolescent. My grandmother and mother carried me as I had to learn how to overcome and conquer testing milestones. I continue to persevere with their wisdom faithfully in life, and I will pass them on through my written testimony. I have immense gratitude for having women like them as my matriarchs.

Being my grandmother's and parent's pride and joy was something I vehemently loved as a child. Yet when I became sick, that feeling instantly disappeared as I fell into a depression and convinced myself that I had failed them. The pain and embarrassment moved swiftly. My grandmother would parade my diagnosis as if it was a badge of honor. I was the "sick one, "she would announce to whoever would listen. Overwhelmed, I sat in silence. At the time, I had just initiated my writing journey solely because I was in between jobs and fresh out of college with a degree in theatre arts and journalism. I would squirm in my chair and smile in embarrassment because I had nothing to show for my degrees or writing skills except diplomas on the living room wall. I wasn't proud of anything I did because I was worried about what I wasn't achieving compared to others my age. "My granddaughter, the writer," she would announce. When asked what I was writing, I would clam up. Before I could formulate a sentence, she would interject, and like the proud Haitian grandmother, she made us endure her awkward game of charades and pointed to her head to interpret my illness as loosely; "a pwoblème ou de Cerveau, "translation: a problem with the brain." She couldn't pronounce Multiple Sclerosis in creole. Then she would gesture the symbol of the cross like a devout Catholic woman and spit three times, damning my diagnosis. She was super Catholic with a bit of superstition balled up in one little lady. She and my mother believed my medical diagnosis made me no less competent nor able to be successful. On the contrary, in my grandmother's eyes, I was more fragile and feebler now than ever, whereas my mother sought my resiliency. My mother and grandmothers' beliefs fueled my journey and faith in how to overcome Multiple Sclerosis.

Introduction

Disclaimer:

It took six years to compile over seventeen years of information and distorted memories, which have grown fuzzier to construct my testimony. Possible side effects from the cocktail of medications I've been prescribed and taken during my lifetime or a symptom from chronic brain inflammation. I also drew from sensory notations and stories told by my grandmother, lovingly known to many as Manmie Lea or Mama Lea, and my mother, Ms. Fanny, which she preferred to be referred to if you were estranged.

I call her Mother dearest or Mommy, as depicted in my cell phone contacts.

My grandmother was sassy, joyful, and inviting. Everyone seemed to call her Mama Lea,

which she embraced. My mother was transparent and bold.

If anyone would dare call her mommy, she will quickly put you in your place and facetiously

reply, "Do I look like your mother?" Then smiled and carried on with whatever she was tending to. My grandmother and mother recounted many of my episodic flare-ups (also known as exacerbations) alongside my one hundred- and sixty pages of medical records. I tried to make the most sense of the pieces I could put together. I spent a decade and a half doing my unbiased research while being placed on various medical therapies. Being a hardheaded pre-teen had its advantages despite its lackluster signs of progress. Through trial and error, I learned to understand, accept my triggers and limitations, draw healthy boundaries, and find immense inner and physical strengths, although it took almost my entire lifetime. My mishaps allowed me to process and learn from my losses and continue to heal time again. Even as the symptoms of Multiple Sclerosis hit my adolescent body, striking like riptides. My mother and grandmother wouldn't allow me to get swept away into the daunting vastness of MS. Every time I needed to start the healing process again, they were present to see me through. My mother kept stern with me. My grandmother wiped away my tears. That wasn't enough.

I researched my way to wellness and overcoming possible death. Not being an actual doctor doesn't place me at any disposition. Yet, my twenty-three years harnessed something more. I feel my experiences should be of access by others, especially young minority children who are left out of the narrative.

I found truth, courage, strength, and discipline and made peace with the harsh realities I acquired along with the battle with the diagnosis. As a child, I only had access to what was given to me, which I still couldn't comprehend. I was fearful and thought that death by disease resulted from my misbehavior. Despite the many times, my parents told me that it wasn't my fault I was sick. I was consumed by negativity and toxicity that it was my fault; consequently, I got sick. During the years, I was pelted with misinformation, lack thereof information, and non-existent representation. Eventually, my grandmother's lessons in faith and my mother's standards kept me focused.

I could omit from time to time the symbiotic relationship Multiple Sclerosis built with my body, but like a shadow, it always lingered. And I would have to succumb to my brutal reality. It became embedded in my life and way of thinking. Regardless, I turned my fears around and used them to fuel my journey. Even though doctors chained me to something, I didn't understand for years, identify with it, or find the need. A diagnosis without a cure made me obsess about my days being numbered so much at such a young age that I couldn't focus on becoming well. I wouldn't be able to rectify anything in my life for years. My health became my mother's and grandmother's strife and struggle more than my own in more instances than one. They spent their lives keeping me alive.

Nothing I could ever do would amount to my parent's and grandmother's sacrifices. The relationship my Manmie Lea and I fostered made my childhood seem magical. Especially pre-diagnosis and in my first two years of misdiagnosis. Our bond was the aesthetics that built what helped me clarify, identify, and simplify the effects Multiple Sclerosis had on my life and how I would learn to cope. My grandmother's prayer and my mother's love fueled me to manifest and work towards a lifestyle that allowed me to learn, adapt and flourish. This malignant autoimmune disease that affects millions around the world is misunderstood by many and is coined the "phantom disease." Living through it for so many years, I understand humanity's shortcomings and inability to come to peace with ourselves. To claim our history and treat our bodies better and be progressive as a unit. Instead, more now than ever, MS has spiked as new cases have been on a steady rise in the black community.

I compiled some essential lessons I've learned to prove how this disease narrative has left out an entire demographic, race, and culture. The records of the young black and brown children have gone undocumented nor given the attention they deserve. Doctors have been gaslighting everything I explained to them. They have tried to silence or push my apprehensions and considered my pain and opinions irrelevant. I was turned into a lab rat, some test subject. They introduced my adolescent body to harmful drugs without offering alternative treatment despite the risks and deadly side effects. I have derived a few of my theories and various conclusions from my first two and a half years of being gaslighted during my wait for a diagnosis.

Medical Biases, Unclarities, and Disparities

Black women and men are marginalized, systemically ostracized, and have dealt with many medical malpractices and oppression. Medically misinformed, misled, misrepresented, and unseen is no longer a standard with chronic and mental illness in the black and brown community. Being oppressed, scared, and scrutinized will be a thing of the past. I am doing my part to use my voice to stop biases of unethical practices and prejudices. I will no longer be bullied into science nor allow myself to be victimized. Being looked at as lesser than humans and discriminated against makes you feel smaller. I guarantee that even though I am not a doctor, we are wiser than doctors give us credit for, but intuitively our bodies can heal from traumas from MS and live a better quality of life. I am a testimony that lifestyle and nutrition are a means to controlling the symptoms of MS.

I am a black woman who had gone through malpractice because of racial iniquities and inequities in the American healthcare system; for years as a child, I couldn't recognize the traumas that were being caused because I didn't know I had a voice. As a child, I was told to listen to and respect adults. I know that it is a community's responsibility to support and make all practical methods available to others and create content to help spread awareness and alternative options.

Diana Lea Maisonenuve is a twenty-five-year Multiple Sclerosis advocate and warrior. Diagnosed with Pediatric Multiple sclerosis at age eight, she was catapulted into a life filled with lessons. She shares her journey with the world to connect and heal others. Her book is broken down into easy-to-read chapters that can guide the reader through her saga, beginning with her unique childhood and relationship with her grandmother. My Tiny Spotted Mind is written to enlighten the next generation of chronic and auto-immune warriors. This is the first book of a trilogy about growing up black in middle America with Multiple Sclerosis. Diana is not only a writer. She has been a thespian since age five, acting in church plays, reciting, writing poetry, and dancing. Join the email list and connect with more like-minded warriors.

Website: MyTinySpottedMind
Instagram: MY TinySpotted Mind
Facebook: Diana Lea

I

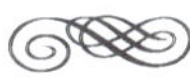

The Old Guitarist

THE OLD GUITARIST

"All I thought I knew was only half of what I needed to understand."-
Diana Lea Maisonneuve

There are parts of history scathed and covered by the ashes of time. Documentation of disease and sickness *are reflected in history for* eons. The wisdom of the "ancient ancestors" were deciphered primarily from outmoded texts filed away in monasteries, pyramids, and libraries, stolen and taken to museums and other verboten institutions. There was the Bronze age, the destruction of Egypt, the fall of Greece, and the demise of the first and second Roman Empires. The over-expansion of Rome led to its downfall and the rise of the largest city of commerce, Constantinople (306-337A.D), now known as Turkey.

During this time, Germanic tribes sacked the Roman empire

multiple times, and finally, it was cited that in 496 A.D, it suffered its death blow. Over a few decades, Europe weakened from the constant raids, and Nordic barbarian tribes destroyed more valuable books and artifacts. It was an ominous tone that flowed through Europe with no innovation or great leaders. Persecution for religious beliefs brought about the rise of Christianity. The crusades (1095 A.D) and rolled out the Medieval times, which lasted till (Mid-1300). Within decades, Europe's significant colonies began to expand into western territories, and wars occurred between kingdoms throughout Europe, leading to millions of deaths. Kingdoms began to explore already inhabited yet undiscovered regions. An Italian sailor named Christopher Columbus was the first to be commissioned by King Ferdinand the second and Queen Isabella of Spain during what ignited the westward expansion. That expansion led Columbus to sail to the warm shores of Hispaniola, present-day Haiti, in 1493. Initially, he was sent on voyages to find a trade route to Asia and stumbled onto indigenous people's shores.

The islands of the Caribbean have been occupied by indigenous people documented since 5000BCE. These villages flourished in 300BCE, with large farming communities claimed by the Arawak group, which became dominant, and Ciboney, which were most prominent. There was also the Taino, the first Arawak people who were also known to be the inhabitants of most of Cuba, Jamaica, Puerto Rico, Haiti, and the Dominican Republic. The islanders based their economy on inter-island trading of cassava, gold, fish, farming, gold- jewelry, pottery, and other goods. After Columbus came to Haiti, the Arawak and Tinos disappeared without a trace. Many sailors would go to the country and never come back. They were establishing a new life on these Islands.

The siege of the Caribbean occurred during a period that unveiled a climate and environment in times of using arbitrary health and hygiene practices that impacted humanity on a global scale. There was much trading by ships that carried goods and merchant seamen in devastating conditions. Columbus began the colonization of Haiti by killing, pillaging, and extracting the island's natural resources for trade. Death and disease began to surge throughout Europe and onwards to the rest of the world. Entanglements between wealth, knowledge, power, religion, and morality impacted mortality and clouded judgment to serve as leverage for cures. Documents left in monasteries remained for interpretation and alluded to superstitions and mystics. A search toward the cosmos for answers fascinated people for decades. There was no distinguished separation between politics and religion. Money bought religious absolution from the church, king, or queen.

Theories and ideologies utilized barbaric methods to cure sickness and disease, leading to the spread of more diseases. Ancient literature was burned in the raiding and looting of the old empires. Destroyed forever within the dwellings of the indigenous peoples' healing practices. They had never faced diseases of this magnitude—illness spreading from one person to another with no cure. Poor sewer systems and hygiene practices amplified the spread of the Black Death, which echoed throughout the world. Medieval times were a heavy and menacing era.

It wasn't until the 19th century, also known as the Victorian Era, that the term "scientist" was coined in 1833 by William Whewell. During that period came a rise of independent researchers such as Darwin and Whewell. The sciences began to flourish by writing books on anatomy, physiology, and biology. All findings before the 19thcentury, physicians didn't have any way to diagnose and identify or verify medical results.

As early as 1838, drawings of autopsies depict what modern-day physicians now recognize as scars in the brain, also known as lesions, and began making clear notations of the abnormalities that have been echoing throughout books since the Middle Ages. Descriptions of the sick were noted but undiagnosed for decades until the 19th century. Autopsies of females that suffered from fits and tremors that were unfamiliar and inconsistent with other cases were compared. Skeptics accused the women of partaking in supernatural nature, demonic possession, sorcery, witchcraft, or other unnatural manifestations and went undiagnosed, left to be tortured, imprisoned, or put to death. Mid to late 19th-century treatment for the occurrences ranged from shock therapy, leeching, imprisonment, or death for those thought to be criminally affiliated. Often, they became the scapegoats for the unjustifiable.

Father of Neurology

Many believe that Jean Martian Charcot was the father of Neurology. To clarify, Charcot was the father of *Modern* Neurology. During my research, I learned that Thomas Willis was the founder of Neurology from 1621-1675. He was a 17th-century English physician and Father of Neuroscience. Willis and his father served during the Civil war because of the family's loyalty to King Charles the 1st. After his parents died, the King recognized young Thomas's services. He then granted him a medical degree in 1646 partly as his loyalty reward. Willis was also a Founder and Fellow of the prestigious Royal Society. He became an essential part of the history of anatomy, psychiatry, and neurology, with famous works focused on nerves and their functions, Neuroscience. Willis used the word "Nero "from the Greek word meaning ligament, tendon, or bowstring.

During the 17th century, the study of anatomy was not understood, and whatever was known was limited. In that era, most of what was known were based on the literature and knowledge of Bergengario, Vesalius, and DaVinci, greatly influenced by the ancient Greek physician Galen. Galen believed that the brain's function was to primarily purify spirits that were blamed for many diseases at the time. He believed in phantom-like spirits or ghosts that could manipulate and make their own decisions. They were responsible for mental disorders such as depression and insanity. The brains that the scientist studied were kept in horrible conditions because they had no effective means to preserve the specimens.

Born in 1825 in France, Jean-Martin Charcot was masterful in the sciences. Because he became fluent in multiple languages, enabling him to pursue various scientific disciplines. He focused on Gerontology, the study of diseases of the joints and lungs, physiology, anatomy of the human body, and pathology. Jean-Martin Charcot ultimately became a professor of Pathological Anatomy at the University of Paris Medicine School. His groundbreaking research on hysteria helped him to gain recognition while studying and during his internship at 'Pitie'- Salpetriere Hospital, which often served as a wasteland for mentally ailed females, vagabonds, and prostitutes. After his training, another revered Neurologist promoted him to the Chef de Clinique, and Charcot returned to Pitie'-Salpetriere Hospital as the senior physician. In 1863, Jean-Martin Charcot was the first to recognize Multiple Sclerosis as a disease. His advancements coined him the father of Neurology.

Charcot utilized his knowledge of his multiple disciplines in science and began examinations on the autopsies of young women suffering from tremors. He introduced photography, ophthalmoscopy, and microcopy at the hospital. During his autopsy, he discovered "Charcot's detailed description of MS" in 1868He continued to describe his observations as *"la sclerosis en plaques"), which were an* accompaniment to the first drawings illustrating the expansions of lesions from the ventricles into the cerebral hemispheres. These detailed sketches depicted the earliest insight into the pathology of MS involving both the brain and spinal cord. He then categorized various forms of MS. He could correlate the symptoms with the findings in the postmortem. Sclerosis meaning' Plaques' or 'many scars' in Latin, accounted for the location of the scars in the MRI. This deterioration happened on the outer nerve covering called the myelin sheath. He observed that his female patients had issues with their speech regarding slurring and dysarthria (default in swallowing), making them inaudible. Most times, patience would choke on their tongues or saliva. He also depicted very abnormally involuntary eye movement and coordination.

.

Hypothesis

Growing up, my experience with Multiple Sclerosis seemed consistent with Charcot's notations and theories. I can sympathize with society's perception and the misinterpretations of people with an invisible illness. Being called every name except my own happened to be expected. Nothing is more unwanted and frustrating than something that makes you feel close to death. It nags at you painfully but doesn't kill you; instead, it makes your life miserable to your very end. Therefore, the methods used to cure most ailments or pain were arbitrary and illogical.

Hot and cold-water baths were one of the tests doctors used to help diagnose MS. It would suggest the relativity of cooler temperatures helped when managing MS symptoms. The hotter and more humid temperatures, the worse symptoms became. Experimental shock therapy and experimental potions were introduced, leading to further handicaps and deaths. Once claimed to be no longer treatable, patients were placed into asylums or left destitute to die in the streets and made out to be social outcasts and lepers. Since the era of Charcot, science and modern technological and medical breakthroughs have brought us closer to treating MS but still no cure. Doctors now use magnetic imaging and rudimentary cognitive and motor tests. Yet MS, because of its bizarre tendencies, is still a combination of a process of elimination and a guessing game.

A series of tests are done, and theories are deduced; the doctors arrive at the MS diagnosis when all other diseases don't match up. My diagnosis jolted my entire family. I understood why people fear what they can't comprehend. I lived in fear for most of my life. I wanted to run away from all my issues because I didn't realize what was happening to me. My lack of awareness and narrow mind fueled my fear and stirred this monster, wreaking havoc inside me. I felt no hope and no clarity on the horizon. My inadequacies and uncertainties kept driving me toward the brink of insanity. I tried to harm myself to stop my body's erratic, spastic, and unearthly impulses.

Multiple Sclerosis struck me like lightning, electrifying my central nervous system and leaving the control center of my body (brain and spinal cord) susceptible to being in incredible amounts of pain or limp. Think of exasperation as a triggered virus in the computer's mainframe that begins attacking itself, trying to rid itself because it identifies as a virus or foreign entity. The chords are wrapped in the protection of rubber coating (myelin sheath), but the layer is eroding and corrupted as the entire internal main frame becomes dysfunctional. On the outside, the computer looks brand new but internally, the computer is scrambled and can't sustain proper function. That's an accurate depiction of how my symptoms with MS have played out.

All my lesions are found in my brain, yet I have had a wide range of symptoms that disrupted my body's internal homeostasis, which caused me cognitive and motor skill disruption. Twitching, drop-foot, and my mouth drooping (Bell's palsy) were among the symptoms that began to ail me. Internally my body was raging war against itself. Fatigue, soreness, spazzing, cramping, tightness in my joints, and brain fog constantly antagonized me and radiated throughout my entire body.

All events after my diagnosis were unforeseen and beyond anyone's immediate control. By age ten, I thought my life was over and figured I would die much sooner than I could fathom. Physically, I bore the pain and burden of an anomaly alone, no matter how much my mother and grandmother tried to soothe my agony. The pains ran rapidly through my body; my mother wouldn't allow me to be less than resilient, for I was to finish whatever I started, especially regarding my academics. That was her bare minimum. Though she was stern, she also was very patient. I didn't understand why she didn't show me any leniency. She maintained our home with such an iron fist.

It took me almost nineteen years to conclude why my mother was strict with me while battling a disease. She wouldn't grant me any leniency. After we had connected with my new neurologist, she took me to every appointment for over twenty years until I moved. I could have sought other options during that time, but I became complacent, and alternatives and other doctors' opinions were unfathomable. We were willing to take any type of answer as long as we could take something that may save my life, which was never guaranteed. Having the same neurologist since I was a child almost made it seem like other doctors were obsolete because of how hard it was to find one to give me an actual diagnosis. Not knowing better immediately eliminated the need to search any further for a second opinion. My mother revered my neurologist so much that I thought solely that the neurologist had the keys to my wellness. Grandmother didn't let up so quickly. Within the first ten years, I learned resiliency and that I had a voice and lived through a unique experience, but I needed to know why. I began journaling and researching rather than becoming dependent on the findings and *expertise* of others. Listen to everything and observe the theories and practices of other auto-compromised "professionals," I investigated the teas and food my grandmother gave me and formulated a plan that worked for me. My first two neurologists never encountered a patient with my circumstances, and I needed answers to my narrative.

It Was All a Dream

In 1999, during the appearance of my first nefarious autoimmune flare, not much was known nor understood about the etymology of Multiple Sclerosis. During my journey, my parents tried to ease my skepticism by not allowing my juvenile brain to form any thoughts or opinions. They were aligned with the doctors prescribed or suggested, and I had no choice. My parents entrusted the neurologist with my life. There was no length my parents wouldn't go to to ensure my lively hood was being looked after. Coming from a Caribbean diaspora, survival was essential. After a temporary residency in two different neurologists' offices, I was approved through my mother's insurance and referred to the only neurologist specializing in pediatric neurology in New York. My family was relieved and saw this as a beacon of light. My grandmother and I believed this was the answer to our prayers. Of course, we did not doubt that they would save me and make this all go away because that was what they were supposed to do.

With a few simple rudimentary cognitive and motor tests, the doctor could tell what was afflicting me was precisely what they had seen in nearly many of their Caucasian patients. The neurologist also noticed issues with y short-term and long-term memory, focus, and information processing. I failed to reach the thresh hold for almost all my motor skills tests. From walking, touching my fingers to my nose, and walking in a straight line like a tightrope, I felt hopeless. On-site neurologist after my first examination, the neurologist confidently diagnosed me with Pediatric Multiple sclerosis (POMS) at age ten.

The final diagnosis left us dumbfounded with questions we may never get the answers to. My mother's signatures and later pamphlets seemed to have sealed my fate. My path began to align with a vastness of mental, physical, and emotional disharmony without any source of direction or accurate explanation of what to expect. I braced myself. I couldn't imagine that things could not get any worse. I have stood corrected many times through my experiences. The thought of diagnosis blindsided me, as I thought a cure was sure to follow. I was expecting it to; we all were. Thus, I began what I considered my MS drug binge. The protocol was to prescribe medicine, then monitor and document its effects. The doctor never told me I had a choice; they just chose for me. Within a week after I began middle school, I was quickly approved for my first medication for MS by my mother's insurance providers. Honestly, the slow maiming experience of MS never seemed more enticing, but once the therapeutics started, so did their adverse effects. The medications harbored notes of illness I had never felt during my weeks in the pediatric care unit.

At random, I would run high fevers. The medications hindered my ability to function normally with society. I tried to keep up with the world around me. During my first trimester of school in the seventh grade, I tried to remain vigilant in my classes. I would intentionally sit in front of the classroom not only to make a good impression but in hopes, I would stay awake and remain attentive to retain that day's lesson plan. I ended up drooling and leaving an embarrassing puddle of saliva on my desk. The teacher or a student would nudge me when I drifted too far off from time to time. It was frustrating because I didn't understand why me. This was unfair. Who or where to place the blame; was this MS or the new drug's side effects? Maybe it was me, and I wasn't trying hard enough. It went beyond my concentration difficulties, insomnia at night, chills, fevers, persistent flu-like symptoms, missed menstrual cycles, twitching and tingling all over my body, and chronic muscle pains. Maybe it was the influx of medications. I didn't fear the drugs; I feared never becoming normal again and failing out of school.

Every time I went to an appointment, I felt apprehension, anxiety, and pressure to medicate. Beyond the fact that I felt as if I was dying, the doctors pelted us with so much information in each appointment that we didn't have time to digest anything, and they warranted an answer at that very moment. There was a lack of transparency, and it was frustrating and stressful. Where one symptom went away, another was there to replace it. My neurologist was ready with every appointment. There was a newer variation of medication, and having options made me rethink my therapies every time I walked into the office. I felt sicker and weaker as my symptoms intensified. I wanted to find a way to stop the pain and run from the madness. Walking out of the office, I was confused, resentful, and angry, with no direction to place my angst. I became aware that my circumstances wouldn't change any time soon and continued to be more willing to accept what I thought would be the end of my life. I was in angst to the point where I wanted to find even more so a cure, not a quick temporary fix with glitches. As I began researching, I learned that the human immune system is designed to protect us from the toxins and harmful bacteria in our environment that may get into our bodies and obstruct our balance. It still didn't make sense; why me? In the case of an autoimmune disease, I wanted to figure out what differentiated me from the other autoimmune-deficient warriors and why there was no cure. I needed to figure out what was making me sick.

Multiple Sclerosis attacks the nervous system cells without warning. The nervous system is a bevy of neurological highway paths ranging from the spinal to the cerebral cortex (brain) and everything between the toes. The presented symptoms should diagnose what autoimmune disease the person has. Unfortunately, some symptoms are so similar that there is often a misdiagnosis or prolonged diagnosis of the disease, which may lead to additional consultations, wrongful medication, and the opinions of several health professionals.

If the MS affects the optical nerves, you must see an eye doctor or optometrist. If it affects your mental health, your neurologist could refer you to a psychologist; your speech will lead you to be referred to a pathologist. I had been referred to none of the above, and this ailment affected me in every single way possible. After I was diagnosed, it felt like the neurologist had opened Pandora's Box filled with prescription medications, endless doctors' appointments, symptoms, and embarrassment. While being transparent and truthful about my symptoms, the doctor kept prescribing more prescription medications. I became depressed and overwhelmed because of the clutter and confusion that sounded to me. Immediately, I was prescribed anti-depressants and pain medications to add to the list. I slowly introduced my body to the pills the doctor prescribed. Other symptoms began to surface, and I started missing more school days. I knew I had to stop taking them, so I hid the prescriptions, hoping my mother would forget because I could no longer tolerate the mood swings, twitching, and migraines. She was distraught when she figured out what I was up to. I told her I couldn't take them anymore. Yet she insisted; therefore, I slipped the pill under my tongue and spat it out when she wasn't looking. Consequently, I began building a high pain threshold because I wanted the doctor to get me off what I saw as unnecessary prescriptions.

Vital Cerebral Information

There are three hundred and fifty neurological conditions in existence. One hundred of them are classified as autoimmune diseases. They range from damage caused to the spine, brain, nerves, and chromosomes. Several neurological conditions can be divided into eighty types of autoimmune diseases. They share similar characteristics. For example, Bell's palsy is associated with the inflammation and swelling of the nerve and muscle that controls the side of the face and jaw, including the mouth. Viral infections and pathogens have also been linked to the development of exacerbations in MS. Bacteria such as Chlamydia pneumonia act as enforcers, also known as superantigens, and viruses, like Epstein-Barr virus and human endogenous retrovirus; the etiology is still unknown. Like many other autoimmune diseases,

MS may be triggered by microbial infections, which is still unknown. Multiple Sclerosis's symptoms mimic fibromyalgia, ALS (Lou Gehrig's disease), Arnold-Chiari deformity, Graves' disease, Stroke, mitochondrial disorders, and Lyme disease, just a few my doctor was able to deduce because all have different prognoses. Their symptoms are close but not identical. Many still display chronic symptoms of some after-effects or trauma, even if they can be cured.

Each prognosis depends on what cells are being attacked, where, how, and what symptoms are experienced. Autoimmune diseases produce antibodies that attract and deteriorate the body's defense system, which starts to operate irrationally and identify healthy cells as foreign cells and tissue. The treatment I was given was steroids to combat the active lesions. I had no say or time to absorb what was happening.

Every medicine is chosen for me after pain and grief rather than alleviation. Scientists often look over the *who because* of a lack of support in healthcare and the representation of black people. Throughout European history, the *who (Caucasians)* had been at the forefront of the medical narrative. Nevertheless, I don't fault science; I fault the people who allow themselves to take The Medical Code of Ethics and aren't here to serve *all* humanity but to suit their pockets. When that happens, our narrative gets overlooked, lost, gaslighted, and we die or become severely handicapped.

MS has the potential to be remissive, progressive, dormant, or aggressive. My symptoms would subside, but the lesions remained active. Doctors spoke about the aggressive inflammation and my nefarious symptoms during routine appointments, which would occur about every three months like clockwork. My symptoms would linger and then be attacked sporadically after my visits and would lessen conveniently during them. I've experienced symptoms from fatigue, fever, numbness, chills, cognitive issues, muscle aches, gut issues, infections, double vision, tremors, lack of balance, and pins and needles, to name a few.

During my research and development, I learned that the medications I was placed on could cause a brain disease called Progressive Multifocal Leukoencephalopathy (PML). It is a virus that damages the brain and leads to sudden death. As my levels remained significantly low for the first few my fear of death remained high. I didn't even understand what PML was, although It came up constantly; no one explained it to my parents or me. After two failed attempts, doctors found a medication that showed promise because of the sustainment of a low PML level. When I began treatment on my third medicine but still sat in agony. I continued to take the medication that we were confident in science would save my life. I was more concerned with how I was supposed to combat my disease, externally knowing there was no cure. No one was worried about my PML but me because I didn't understand what it was, among other things the doctors spoke about. I couldn't understand the side effects that treatment could have on my body nor what else MS had in store for me at such a young age, so I kept following doctors' orders hoping my symptoms would be alleviated and I would recover. Doctors mostly spoke around me, not directly to me, unless it was about dosages for medicine and how to inject myself.

Whatever was transpiring inside my brain was killing me from all sides. We all wanted me fixed. My flares presumably turned into full relapse after relapse with small spurts of remission, which caused me immense pain. I didn't understand how to keep my symptoms under control. Each therapy came with many side effects that I would never be able to tame at such a young age. Again, I was uncertain if it was the medicine of the MS. I tried to sleep away the pain as much as possible. Even if I wasn't tired. Many of the times, it was against my will anyway. Most nights, I was an insomniac, and when it came to the day, my fatigue would turn me into a zombie.

I think these treatments aimed to help the patients maintain and stabilize remission so that the flares won't lead to further handicaps. Like an autoimmune disease, the point is to be in remission for life, meaning no abnormal brain activity. My symptoms would disappear and come back full throttle, even in different forms of pain. I believe and hope humanity can agree that remissions are true miracles. I just couldn't find my advantage.

It took me years to come to terms with and find a place where I felt comfortable confiding in anyone, let alone my parents, doctors, or even opening the world. My mother adjusted to the news of my diagnosis in her way. She was never an openly emotional person. Powerful indeed, willed, witty, and blunt. When company came over for dinner parties, she would broadcast my diagnosis as an introduction that I was present in the room. MS quickly became my plus one. As I walked into the room, she presented me as she explained, and I followed. I felt their eyes burning through my skin. The standard was to say good evening, "Bonsoir," to every guest in the room. I was fighting an incurable chronic disease and quickly became the elephant in the room. Then she told me to pronounce the medication I was taking. As if anyone understood what we were talking about because we weren't aware of what I was up against. I guess that was her way of dealing with my disease. Being proud of the strength she thought I had because she expected it from me.

My grandmother, on the other hand, indulged me and held me close. Although, I was unhappy with how she dealt with the information similarly. Gesturing to her head as her eyes began swelling up with tears. I would smile painfully and try to respectfully remove myself from any further ridicule or multitudes of questions. Once the fact that I was ill was brought up, guests berated me with awkward and intense questions and energy.

I didn't know how to answer, nor was I willing to explain what I didn't understand. I wanted to shrink and wither away. A heavy feeling loomed over my body, my chest compressed tightly, and my alms would sweat profusely. I became riddled with anxiety. So, I wittingly broke away and excused myself. I would mention that I needed to go to bed early because of school. I felt terrible when I did because I wasn't tired; instead, I was embarrassed and infuriated with my mother and grandmother for announcing and brandishing my misery and vulnerability amongst their guests. I became my own Achilles heel because of the emotions I began to develop internally. I started to horde and filled myself with animosity despite how much love I was being given; nothing seemed enough to extinguish the overwhelming feeling of embarrassment and angst. I started to second guess everyone's intention toward me, beginning with my parents. Why was it anyone's business? Did they have a cure? No one cared nor could understand what I was going through. I felt as if I was being made out to be a spectacle.

I realized much later in life that nothing I have ever felt nor am feeling was wrong or should be taken lightly. Just because you can't see it doesn't mean it doesn't exist or matter. Inside my body, war was beginning to erupt, and I wasn't equipped for the fight of my life, especially if I wanted a runaway from my circumstances. Although I knew it wasn't my mother's fault, I held a grudge fueled by hatred and fear. Yet, in the back of my mind, my intuition told me she might have been doing all she could. Mentally, spiritually, and emotionally needed to resolve a problem I could not comprehend.

People would stare blankly and say, *"wow, you don't look like you're sick."*. I couldn't make sense of their choice of words when I felt as if life was slipping from me. I hated my existence. They often made me feel like I was lying, which confused my adolescent mind. Months passed, and I still couldn't accept what I didn't understand. My inevitable of being this broken brown girl, constantly struggling to climb up the downward spiraling ladder of health in a society where we aren't taught about health and wellness. At one point, I thought that they would eventually disappear if I ignored the symptoms. After my diagnosis and learning that there was no cure, MS became my lifelong fight. I would be hammered with therapies and side effects. The American dream seemed unreal because of my lack of knowledge and awareness. I didn't think my body would ever be able again. I thought I would have to accept whatever was to come. My idea of happily ever after seemed bleak.

I give no disease any hierarchy over the other. I speak solely through my own experiences. This book is written to raise awareness among children with autoimmune diseases and the black Multiple Sclerosis community. I hope everyone can finish this book and find vital information between its pages. I am giving a face and a voice to the unheard and amplifying the wellness and mental health within the black community. I once was ashamed to identify with Multiple Sclerosis, not just because it made me different, but because I was scared, alone, and ill-equipped to fight. I cycled medicines until my body rejected them one after another, praying the next drug would have fewer symptoms. There is blatant discord in the black narrative, especially for children of color. Bringing awareness to this narrative helped me persevere through my pain and write this book while working a full-time job and my wellness.

It took me almost fifteen years to finally realize that I wouldn't die from Multiple Sclerosis despite what I was told or how much pain I was in. Instead, I could die from the medications' because they may cause further complications. I feel that humanity is forced into such conformity of *quick fixes*. After being told I had a disease, one option was presented to me. My juvenile mind immediately associated my diagnosis with death; the medication was what was my glimpse of hope until I figured out its catastrophic side effects. If you follow the flow, you will end up adrift and disillusioned. I was once confused and almost lost touch with reality. I didn't understand that my diagnosis wasn't my identity. My lack of knowledge was me walking down death row.

Though the timing is everything, it took me quite a while to find my courage and allow myself to heal and find my safe place. I continue to reflect and research feverously during my quest for change in the de-marginalization and systemic oppression of health care for black people and a cure for Multiple pediatric Sclerosis.

Hypothesis

As a child, my experience with Multiple Sclerosis seemed consistent with Charcot's notations and theories. I can sympathize with society's perception and the misinterpretations of people with an invisible illness. Being called every name except my own happened to be expected. Nothing is more unwanted and frustrating than something that makes you feel close to death. It nags at you painfully but doesn't kill you; instead, it makes your life miserable to your very end. Therefore, the methods used to cure most ailments or pain were arbitrary and illogical.

Hot and cold-water baths were one of the tests doctors used to help diagnose MS. It would suggest the relativity of cooler temperatures helped when managing MS symptoms. The hotter and more humid temperatures, the worse symptoms became. Experimental shock therapy and experimental potions were introduced, leading to further handicaps and deaths. Once claimed to be no longer treatable, patients were placed into asylums or left destitute to die in the streets and made out to be social outcasts and lepers. Since the era of Charcot, science and modern technological and medical breakthroughs have brought us closer to treating MS but still no cure. Doctors now use magnetic imaging and rudimentary cognitive and motor tests. Yet MS, because of its bizarre tendencies, is still a combination of a process of elimination and a guessing game.

A series of tests are done, and theories are deduced; the doctors arrive at the MS diagnosis when all other diseases don't match up. My diagnosis jolted my entire family. I understood why people fear what they can't comprehend. I lived in fear for most of my life. I wanted to run away from all my issues because I didn't realize what was happening to me. My lack of awareness and narrow mind fueled my fear and stirred this monster, wreaking havoc inside me. I felt no hope and no clarity on the horizon. My inadequacies and uncertainties kept driving me toward the brink of insanity. I tried to harm myself to stop my body's erratic, spastic, and unearthly impulses.

Multiple Sclerosis struck me like lightning, electrifying my central nervous system and leaving the control center of my body (brain and spinal cord) susceptible to being in incredible amounts of pain or limp. Think of exasperation as a triggered virus in the computer's mainframe that begins attacking itself, trying to rid itself because it identifies as a virus or foreign entity. The chords are wrapped in the protection of rubber coating (myelin sheath), but the layer is eroding and corrupted as the entire internal main frame becomes dysfunctional. On the outside, the computer looks brand new but internally, the computer is scrambled and can't sustain proper function. That's an accurate depiction of how my symptoms with MS have played out.

All my lesions are found in my brain, yet I have had a wide range of symptoms that disrupted my body's internal homeostasis, which caused me cognitive and motor skill disruption. Twitching, drop-foot, and my mouth drooping (Bell's palsy) were among the symptoms that began to ail me. Internally my body was raging war against itself. Fatigue, soreness, spazzing, cramping, tightness in my joints, and brain fog constantly antagonized me and radiated throughout my entire body.

All events after my diagnosis were unforeseen and beyond anyone's immediate control. By age ten, I thought my life was over and figured I would die much sooner than I could fathom. Physically, I bore the pain and burden of an anomaly alone, no matter how much my mother and grandmother tried to soothe my agony. The pains ran rapidly through my body; my mother wouldn't allow me to be less than resilient, for I was to finish whatever I started, especially regarding my academics. That was her bare minimum. Though she was stern, she also was very patient. I didn't understand why she didn't show me any leniency. She maintained our home with such an iron fist.

It took me almost nineteen years to conclude why my mother was strict with me while battling a disease. She wouldn't grant me any leniency. After we had connected with my new neurologist, she took me to every appointment for over twenty years until I moved. I could have sought other options during that time, but I became complacent, and alternatives and other doctors' opinions were unfathomable. We were willing to take any type of answer as long as we could take something that may save my life, which was never guaranteed. Having the same neurologist since I was a child almost made it seem like other doctors were obsolete because of how hard it was to find one to give me an actual diagnosis. Not knowing better immediately eliminated the need to search any further for a second opinion. My mother revered my neurologist so much that I thought solely that the neurologist had the keys to my wellness. Grandmother didn't let up so quickly. Within the first ten years, I learned resiliency and that I had a voice and lived through a unique experience, but I needed to know why. I began journaling and researching rather than becoming dependent on the findings and *expertise* of others. Listen to everything and observe the theories and practices of other auto-compromised "professionals," I investigated the teas and food my grandmother gave me and formulated a plan that worked for me. My first two neurologists never encountered a patient with my circumstances, and I needed answers to my narrative.

It Was All a Dream

In 1999, during the appearance of my first nefarious autoimmune flare, not much was known nor understood about the etymology of Multiple Sclerosis. During my journey, my parents tried to ease my skepticism by not allowing my juvenile brain to form any thoughts or opinions. They were aligned with the doctors prescribed or suggested, and I had no choice. My parents entrusted the neurologist with my life. There was no length my parents wouldn't go to to ensure my lively hood was being looked after. Coming from a Caribbean diaspora, survival was essential. After a temporary residency in two different neurologists' offices, I was approved through my mother's insurance and referred to the only neurologist specializing in pediatric neurology in New York. My family was relieved and saw this as a beacon of light. My grand-mother and I believed this was the answer to our prayers. Of course, we did not doubt that they would save me and make this all go away because that was what they were supposed to do.

With a few simple rudimentary cognitive and motor tests, the doctor could tell what was afflicting me was precisely what they had seen in nearly many of their Caucasian patients. The neurologist also noticed issues with y short-term and long-term memory, focus, and information processing. I failed to reach the thresh hold for almost all my motor skills tests. From walking, touching my fingers to my nose, and walking in a straight line like a tightrope, I felt hopeless. On-site neurologist after my first examination, the neurologist confidently diagnosed me with Pediatric Multiple sclerosis (POMS) at age ten.

The final diagnosis left us dumbfounded with questions we may never get the answers to. My mother's signatures and later pamphlets seemed to have sealed my fate. My path began to align with a vastness of mental, physical, and emotional disharmony without any source of direction or accurate explanation of what to expect. I braced myself. I couldn't imagine that things could not get any worse. I have stood corrected many times through my experiences. The thought of diagnosis blindsided me, as I thought a cure was sure to follow. I was expecting it to; we all were. Thus, I began what I considered my MS drug binge. The protocol was to prescribe medicine, then monitor and document its effects. The doctor never told me I had a choice; they just chose for me. Within a week after I began middle school, I was quickly approved for my first medication for MS by my mother's insurance providers. Honestly, the slow maiming experience of MS never seemed more enticing, but once the therapeutics started, so did their adverse effects. The medications harbored notes of illness I had never felt during my weeks in the pediatric care unit.

I began becoming feverish randomly. The medications hindered my ability to function normally with society. I tried to keep up with the world around me. During my first trimester of school in the seventh grade, I tried to remain vigilant in my classes. I would intentionally sit in front of the classroom not only to make a good impression but in hopes, I would stay awake and remain attentive to retain that day's lesson plan. I ended up drooling and leaving an embarrassing puddle of saliva on my desk. The teacher or a student would nudge me when I drifted too far off from time to time. It was frustrating because I didn't understand why me. This was unfair. Who or where to place the blame; was this MS or the new drug's side effects? Maybe it was me, and I wasn't trying hard enough. It went beyond my concentration difficulties, insomnia at night, chills, fevers, persistent flu-like symptoms, missed menstrual cycles, twitching and tingling all over my body, and chronic muscle pains. Maybe it was the influx of medications. I didn't fear the drugs; I feared never becoming normal again and failing out of school.

Every time I went to an appointment, I felt apprehension, anxiety, and pressure to medicate. Beyond the fact that I felt as if I was dying, the doctors pelted us with so much information in each appointment that we didn't have time to digest anything, and they warranted an answer at that very moment. There was a lack of transparency, and it was frustrating and stressful. Where one symptom went away, another was there to replace it. My neurologist was ready with every appointment. There was a newer variation of medication, and having options made me rethink my therapies every time I walked into the office. I felt sicker and weaker as my symptoms intensified. I wanted to find a way to stop the pain and run from the madness. Walking out of the office, I was confused, resentful, and angry, with no direction to place my angst. I became aware that my circumstances wouldn't change any time soon and continued to be more willing to accept what I thought would be the end of my life. I was in angst to the point where I wanted to find even more so a cure, not a quick temporary fix with glitches. As I began researching, I learned that the human immune system is designed to protect us from the toxins and harmful bacteria in our environment that may get into our bodies and obstruct our balance. It still didn't make sense; why me? In the case of an autoimmune disease, I wanted to figure out what differentiated me from the other autoimmune-deficient warriors and why there was no cure. I needed to figure out what was making me sick.

Multiple Sclerosis attacks the nervous system cells without warning. The nervous system is a bevy of neurological highway paths ranging from the spinal to the cerebral cortex (brain) and everything between the toes. The presented symptoms should diagnose what autoimmune disease the person has. Unfortunately, some symptoms are so similar that there is often a misdiagnosis or prolonged diagnosis of the disease, which may lead to additional consultations, wrongful medication, and the opinions of several health professionals.

If the MS affects the optical nerves, you must see an eye doctor or optometrist. If it affects your mental health, your neurologist could refer you to a psychologist; your speech will lead you to be referred to a pathologist. I had been referred to none of the above, and this ailment affected me in every single way possible. After I was diagnosed, it felt like the neurologist had opened Pandora's Box filled with prescription medications, endless doctors' appointments, symptoms, and embarrassment. While being transparent and truthful about my symptoms, the doctor kept prescribing more prescription medications. I became depressed and overwhelmed because of the clutter and confusion that sounded to me. Immediately, I was prescribed anti-depressants and pain medications to add to the list. I slowly introduced my body to the pills the doctor prescribed. Other symptoms began to surface, and I started missing more school days. I knew I had to stop taking them, so I hid the prescriptions, hoping my mother would forget because I could no longer tolerate the mood swings, twitching, and migraines. She was distraught when she figured out what I was up to. I told her I couldn't take them anymore. Yet she insisted; therefore, I slipped the pill under my tongue and spat it out when she wasn't looking. Consequently, I began building a high pain threshold because I wanted the doctor to get me off what I saw as unnecessary prescriptions.

Vital Cerebral Information

There are three hundred and fifty neurological conditions in existence. One hundred of them are classified as autoimmune diseases. They range from damage caused to the spine, brain, nerves, and chromosomes. Several neurological conditions can be divided into eighty types of autoimmune diseases. They share similar characteristics. For example, Bell's palsy is associated with the inflammation and swelling of the nerve and muscle that controls the side of the face and jaw, including the mouth. Viral infections and pathogens have also been linked to the development of exacerbations in MS. Bacteria such as Chlamydia pneumonia act as enforcers, also known as superantigens, and viruses, like Epstein-Barr virus and human endogenous retrovirus; the etiology is still unknown. Like many other autoimmune diseases, MS may be triggered by microbial infections, which is still unknown. Multiple Sclerosis's symptoms mimic fibromyalgia, ALS (Lou Gehrig's disease), Arnold-Chiari deformity, Graves' disease, Stroke, mitochondrial disorders, and Lyme disease, just a few my doctor was able to deduce because all have different prognoses. Their symptoms are close but not identical. Many still display chronic symptoms of some after-effects or trauma, even if they can be cured.

Each prognosis depends on what cells are being attacked, where, how, and what symptoms are experienced. Autoimmune diseases produce antibodies that attract and deteriorate the body's defense system, which starts to operate irrationally and identify healthy cells as foreign cells and tissue. The treatment I was given was steroids to combat the active lesions. I had no say or time to absorb what was happening.

Every medicine is chosen for me after pain and grief rather than alleviation. Scientists often look over the *who because* of a lack of support in healthcare and the representation of black people. Throughout European history, the *who (Caucasians)* had been at the forefront of the medical narrative. Nevertheless, I don't fault science; I fault the people who allow themselves to take The Medical Code of Ethics and aren't here to serve *all* humanity but to suit their pockets. When that happens, our narrative gets overlooked, lost, gaslighted, and we die or become severely handicapped.

MS has the potential to be remissive, progressive, dormant, or aggressive. My symptoms would subside, but the lesions remained active. Doctors spoke about the aggressive inflammation and my nefarious symptoms during routine appointments, which would occur about every three months like clockwork. My symptoms would linger and then be attacked sporadically after my visits and would lessen conveniently during them. I've experienced symptoms from fatigue, fever, numbness, chills, cognitive issues, muscle aches, gut issues, infections, double vision, tremors, lack of balance, and pins and needles, to name a few.

During my research and development, I learned that my medication could cause a brain disease called Progressive Multifocal Leukoencephalopathy (PML). It is a virus that damages the brain and leads to sudden death. My levels remained low for quite a few months with the medication I was on. After two failed attempts, this medication showed promise because of the sustainment of a low PML level, but I was in agony while on it. I continued to take the medication that we were confident would save my life. I was more concerned with how I was supposed to combat my disease, knowing there was no cure. No one was worried about my PML. I couldn't understand the side effects that treatment could have on my body nor what else MS had in store for me at such a young age, so I kept following doctors' orders hoping my symptoms would be alleviated and I would recover.

Whatever was transpiring inside my brain was killing me from all sides. We all wanted me fixed. My flares presumably turned into full relapse after relapse with small spurts of remission, which caused me immense pain. I didn't understand how to keep my symptoms under control. Each therapy came with many side effects that I would never be able to tame at such a young age. Again, I was uncertain if it was the medicine of the MS. I tried to sleep away the pain as much as possible. Even if I wasn't tired. Many of the times, it was against my will anyway. Most nights, I was an insomniac, and when it came to the day, my fatigue would turn me into a zombie.

I think these treatments aimed to help the patients maintain and stabilize remission so that the flares won't lead to further handicaps. Like an autoimmune disease, the point is to be in remission for life, meaning no abnormal brain activity. My symptoms would disappear and come back full throttle, even in different forms of pain. I believe and hope humanity can agree that remissions are true miracles. I just couldn't find my advantage.

It took me years to come to terms with and find a place where I felt comfortable confiding in anyone, let alone my parents or doctors. My mother adjusted to the news of my diagnosis in her way. She was never an openly emotional person. Powerful indeed, willed, witty, and blunt. When company came over for dinner parties, she would broadcast my diagnosis as an introduction that I was present in the room. MS quickly became my plus one. As I walked into the room, she presented me as she explained, and I followed. I felt their eyes burning through my skin. The standard was to say good evening, "Bonsoir," to every guest in the room. I was fighting an incurable chronic disease and quickly became the elephant in the room. Then she told me to pronounce the medication I was taking. As if anyone understood what we were talking about because we weren't aware of what I was up against. I guess that was her way of dealing with my disease. Being proud of the strength she thought I had because she expected it from me.

My grandmother, on the other hand, coddled me and held me close. Although, I was unhappy with how she dealt with the information similarly. Gesturing to her head as her eyes began swelling up with tears. I would watch and smile painfully. Try to remain respectful as I remove myself from further ridicule or multitudes of questions. Once the fact that I was ill was brought up, guests berated me with awkward and intense questions and energy.

I didn't know how to answer, nor was I willing to explain what I didn't understand. I wanted to shrink and wither away. A heavy feeling loomed over my body, my chest compressed tightly, and my alms would sweat profusely. I became riddled with anxiety. So, I wittingly broke away and excused myself. I would mention that I needed to go to bed early because of school. I felt terrible when I did because I wasn't tired; instead, I was embarrassed and infuriated with my mother and grandmother for announcing and brandishing my misery and vulnerability amongst their guests. I became my own Achilles heel because of the emotions I began to develop internally. I started to horde and filled myself with animosity despite how much love I was being given; nothing seemed enough to extinguish the overwhelming feeling of embarrassment and angst. I started to second guess everyone's intention toward me, beginning with my parents. Why was it anyone's business? Did they have a cure? No one cared nor could understand what I was going through. I felt as if I was being made out to be a spectacle.

I realized much later in life that nothing I have ever felt nor am feeling was wrong or should be taken lightly. Just because you can't see it doesn't mean it doesn't exist or matter. Inside my body, war was beginning to erupt, and I wasn't equipped for the fight of my life, especially if I wanted a runaway from my circumstances. Although I knew it wasn't my mother's fault, I held a grudge fueled by hatred and fear. Yet, in the back of my mind, my intuition told me she might have been doing all she could. Mentally, spiritually, and emotionally needed to resolve a problem I could not comprehend.

People would stare blankly and say, *"wow, you don't look like you're sick."*. I couldn't make sense of their choice of words when I felt as if life was slipping from me. I hated my existence. They often made me feel like I was lying, which confused my adolescent mind. Months passed, and I still couldn't accept what I didn't understand. My inevitable of being this broken brown girl started to become my constant. I was constantly struggling to climb up the downward spiraling ladder of health in a society where we aren't taught about health and wellness. At one point, I thought that they would eventually disappear if I ignored the symptoms. After my diagnosis and learning that there was no cure, MS became my forever fight. I would be bettered with therapies and their side effects. The American dream seemed unreal because of my lack of knowledge and awareness. I didn't think my body would ever be able again. I thought I would have to accept whatever was to come. My idea of happily ever after seemed bleak.

I give no disease any hierarchy over the other. I speak solely through my own experiences. This book is written to raise awareness among children with autoimmune diseases and the black Multiple Sclerosis community. I hope everyone can finish this book and find vital information between its pages. I am giving a face and a voice to the unheard and amplifying the wellness and mental health within the black community. I once was ashamed to identify with Multiple Sclerosis, not just because it made me different, but because I was scared, alone, and ill-equipped to fight. I cycled medicines until my body rejected them one after another, praying the next drug would have fewer symptoms. There is blatant discord in the black narrative, especially for children of color. Bringing awareness to this narrative helped me persevere through my pain and write this book while working a full-time job and my wellness.

It took me almost fifteen years to finally realize that I wouldn't die from Multiple Sclerosis despite what I was told or how much pain I was in. Instead, I could die from the medications' because they may cause further complications. I feel that humanity is forced into such conformity of *quick fixes*. After being told I had a disease, one option was presented to me. My juvenile mind immediately associated my diagnosis with death; the medication was what was my glimpse of hope until I figured out its catastrophic side effects. If you follow the flow, you will end up adrift and disillusioned. I was once confused and almost lost touch with reality. I didn't understand that my diagnosis wasn't my identity. My lack of knowledge was me walking down death row.

Though the timing is everything, it took me quite a while to find my courage and allow myself to heal and find my safe place. An ability that cant be given to you but one has to find within their faith and themselves. I continue to reflect and research feverously during my quest for change in the demarginalization and systemic oppression of health care for black people and a cure for Multiple pediatric Sclerosis.

2

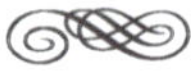

So, Child Like – "The Dream"

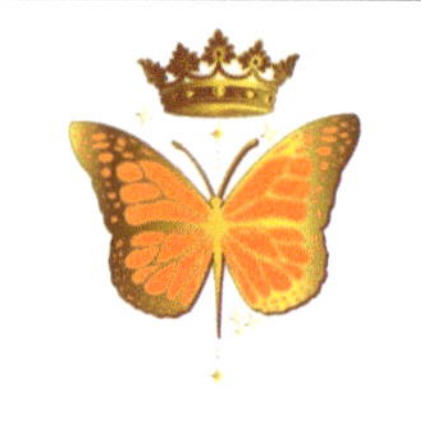

"Every child is an artist. The problem is to remain an artist once they grow up."- Pablo Picasso

I am a first-generation Haitian American woman. My mother moved from Haiti to New York as a young, divorced mother of two to provide her mother and children with better opportunities. My mother left Haiti in the eighties to build a safe lifestyle and evade the political unrest and corruption during the Duvalier dynasty. She made the difficult decision to move to America, leaving behind my older siblings, Stephanie and Sacha. My mother was the second oldest of five children my grandmother birthed. They remained in Haiti with their godparents as she and Manmie Lea became acclimated to America.

I was told my sibling's caretaker was more than stern and less than a kind woman. Still, under the circumstances, my mother left Stephanie and Sacha to be well taken care of and continued their private schooling as she transitioned to the United States. My mother and grandmother had difficulty being far from the kids. One day my brother called them in tears. My mother had enough and, at once, urgently sent for them in fear that her children were being neglected and mistreated. My grandmother, mother, brother, and sister spent a few months cohabitating with my aunt. Fourteen years older than my mother, my aunt had married a suave regal businessman. She lived in a lovely home on Long Island, New York, and was raising three kids. My mother looked at my aunt's husband almost as a father figure; he was twice her age.

With my aunt's and uncle's assistance, my mother gained traction in American economics at a cost. My mom quickly realized that nothing in America was free. My mother's nativity was costly, and she grew wisdom and resilience through disappointment. She wasted no time removing herself from a less favorable environment within a year after she witnessed crude and cruel behavior from her brother-in-law towards my aunt. By then, she was ready to cut ties with my aunt and uncle because there was much disrespect, and she refused to endure the toxicity. She moved out, taking Manama Lea and the children. I moved into an apartment in queens. Jean, my father, whom she married and later moved in. My parents were very ambitious and wanted to build a home. My mother told me that within two years, she got pregnant with me and continued to work almost to full term, regardless of doctors' orders. For my mother, there was no slowing down.

My family enjoyed taking road trips to see distant family. It was amidst their travels to Boston, Massachusetts, while visiting my father's brother, she gave birth to me via c-section at Cambridge hospital. As onlookers watched, my parents' aspirations continued to grow, as my mother had already put in motion that in her return to New York, she would be working. Their sights were set on transitioning from an apartment into a house. My mother was always willing to make the necessary sacrifices to achieve what many believed to be unattainable. They persevered and provided us with everything money had to offer.

They were baby boomers that progressed through the eighties; infused with racism and the ominous crack era, they preserved and persevered through all stigmas against them. Every decade, something was always amidst, trying to stop and divide the success of the structure of the black family. Despite financial and socioeconomic obstacles, my parents remained diligent and focused on building a foundation. Their trilingual tongues and less-than-perfect English skills opened the door to opportunities for themselves to grant us a comfortable lifestyle. The transition to middle-class America was filled with struggles. Their less-than-perfect English skills would slowly become the primary language of the household, and native tongues and dialects would be replaced.

My parents purchased their first home in nineteen eighty-nine; I had just turned three. We were in the same town as my aunt in Long Island, New York. My parents worked feverously. As a unit, they kept a solid roof over our heads, clothes on our backs, and food on the table. My father became their father as much as he was mine. I was unaware that we had different fathers until my late teens, which didn't waiver my love or respect for them.

When I was conceived, my grandmother was seventy years young. She mirrored the appearance of a forty-year-old lady in waiting, for she had no husband, nor was she waiting for one. She had no desire to be wed after my belated grandfather passed; she then devoted the rest of her life to her children and God. Time was very generous to my grandmother's appearance, and she wore her age with such style, grace, and sincerity that no one knew my grandmother's actual age except for whatever age she gave on her passport. Manmie Lea, as her friends and family referred to her, had skin the color of caramel and didn't have a wrinkle. Manmie Lea looked flawlessly ageless. She was kind as she was stunningly timeless. Her hair felt like freshly woven silk, and its color was auburn red. She carried the spirit of a teenager. She was very whimsical, youthful, candid, and free-spirited.

Along with the wisdom of Gandhi and had a heart warm and soulful like Aretha. Manmie Lea harvested a sharp blade-like tong like a sailor. Amazingly candid and sensitive, covered in sass.

Even though the curse words weren't in English, no matter what walk of life, you came from, all would enjoy her audacious humor. French or Creole; her spirit was out of this world and skillfully inappropriate. She was animated, funny, and joyful, yet still coquette. She quickly became everyone's grandmother and the life of the party and every family gathering. Mama Lea, known to many, cared for and fed everyone with overflowing love and the most delicious food. Manmie Lea's food provided everyone comfort, reassurance, and nourishment.

Time Well Spent

Manmie Lea was an amazingly unique, nurturing matriarch. I was practically raised in her arms. I learned French and Creole because It was necessary for our communication. She never bothered to learn how to drive or speak much English, partly stifling her communication ability; therefore, I became her translator. She was very amicable and warm; her divine energy and spirit made it easy for her to form bonds with others. My grandmother was a vivacious God-fearing woman. She began to teach me how to read the Bible in French and Creole.

Manmie Lea and I spent a lot of quality time together, sometimes in the backyard of my home for hours during most seasons. She didn't mind New York's heat or humidity because she was born in Haiti's fiery climate. She never entirely adjusted to the winters in New York, but she endured them without complaint because she was with the love of her children and grandchildren. My family's adjustment to four seasons was a bit rough for them. Regardless of being born on the east coast, I learned I would have the most challenging time. Many of our winters in New York were filled with tall snowfalls and icy and ferocious winds. We spent our days outdoors in late spring, summer, and early fall. Manmie Lea spent lots of time teaching me how to garden. We would plant vegetables and herbs. We picked fresh peppers, mint, thyme, cucumbers, eggplant, basil, zucchini, tomatoes, and other spices. I would eat them straight off the vine. She would put them in the food she cooked and brewed fresh tea.

After picking ingredients from our garden, I followed her in, excited to see what dish she was conjuring up. I stood by, watching her finesse the food with intent and love. She danced in the kitchen in heels most mornings after church, singing and praising while cooking up a feast.

All who knew her enjoyed her humor, charisma, candid energy, and cooking in one breath. Her culinary skills stemmed from her youth when she earned the title of "Le Cordon Bleu," a master's in culinary arts. In Haiti, she was a chef for affluent families all over the country. Her love of nurturing others was beautiful. She always wanted to cook for guests insisting that they were hungry. Pouring her heart into her cooking made her meals even more delicious. Loving to serve her guests, she would set a placemat with the cutlery, a knife on the left-hand side, a fork and spoon on the other, and a folded napkin seated under a glass of drinking water with ice. Grams was majestic, even when she brought me soup on a tray when I wasn't feeling well. I picked up how to cook, clinging to her side as she spent hours preparing daily. *I wish I could hold on to her tighter*, absorbing her every lesson.

Often my attention would veer off into the backyard. During cooking intermissions, she would take me on walks around the yard or hang out in the garden. I would admire the airplanes one by one flying overhead. We resided no less than fifteen minutes from John F. Kennedy Airport. I innately became enamored with planes. I would dance around and shout airplane, she would look at me puzzled, and then I would point to the sky. She would look up and tell me too, say in French, "*avion*," then I would repeat after her, "avions!" as we watched the airplanes fly by. I loved traveling with my grandmother. I remember how massive their aircraft was, taking us to a place that felt like this magic and comfort.

My backyard seemed so grand. It was my magic garden. I enjoyed the outdoors, and my mother was extremely overprotective, so much so that my mother orchestrated a massive fence to be built with a large green awning to shield the backyard. Soon after, our father brought my older sister a Rottweiler/ German Shepard. She named him Jordan after the greatest basketball player of my time. Jorden, within three years, would tower over my father, who was six foot two. There would be no one in and out of our gate. Jorden was my part-time horse. When the weather was inclement, I still enjoyed the outdoors under the awning my mother built over our side yard and playing with the puppy. I would hide from the rain under it during the summer or spring showers. Somedays, I would run amuck indoors when being outdoors wasn't possible. I enjoyed twirling, dancing, and doing cartwheels around the house in song. My favorite activity was dancing and traveling with Manmie Lea, hands down.

I drove Sacha and Stephanie up the wall. I wanted their undivided attention when grandma and our parents weren't around. I wouldn't stop until I had it because I needed my audience. Once I had them seated, the rest of my audience filled in, including some characters I scribbled out of random scrap paper from their school projects and a few of my favorite plush toys. Mom never let the dog sit in. I threw tantrums until my grandmother walked in, or my brother and sister would start singing and clapping their hands to turn my attention away from our puppy, Jordan. He was a German Shepard and my teddy bear. I soon lost interest and would ramble stories or dance around in circles until I was sleepy. Grandma Lea would walk into the living room or den ever so often and not only check on us but also dance along, shaking her hips and enabling me. When my siblings had enough of my overzealous energy, they would try to end my encore, which I cheered on until I would be rushed off to hang out with my grandmother in the kitchen.

We would continue to dance and sing with me tirelessly until I built up a good appetite. Manmie Lea couldn't handle my hyper and curious energy all the time. It got me into trouble- which she couldn't always help me get out of. I would want to play hide and seek conveniently at bedtime. My tiny frame allowed me to fit into just about everywhere.

My childhood home was made up of seven bedrooms. I would hide so well; I found Narnia before there was such a thing. My family had to childproof our home often because I would find new ways to get into things.

Then I would have dinner, bathed and coddled, and off to bed. I always felt safe with her.

My grandmother was my cheerleader.

Manmie Lea was vital to developing and retaining my cultural and spiritual heritage. Although she raised me to be aware of my culture, no history was written. Everything was passed down through word of mouth. She continued traditions and gifted me with morals and a deep reverence for God. Within a short time, Manmie Lea and I fostered an inseparable bond. She became my companion. We would cook, travel, and attend Catholic mass together. We were adjoined at the hip. My middle name was gifted to me by her to honor her as our matriarch. Wherever she went, I wanted to go.

Regardless of what things I could get myself into, I knew there wasn't anything my smile couldn't get me out of. After several unending minutes of hiding and seek, my siblings would finally find me, and all I would do was giggle and toss them a smile and shrug. They would fall into the bad potholes God embedded on each side of my face. My dimples were deep to the point that my family would love to poke my cheeks, and I would be acquitted. There was no harm I could do. I was the baby for the time and reveled in my place.

My childhood was full of wonder and happiness—the joy you see in a child's eyes. Being the first child between my mother and father and the new addition to my family in ten years, they treated me like a mahogany porcelain baby doll. My sister would dress me in pretty bows and matching Air Jordans' and carry me around. Filled with the brownest melanin and a deep golden undertone, I was assertive in my skin because of the love of my sibling's security that my grandmother and mother instilled in me. I wanted to be fearless like them. I viewed them as the epitome of beauty. They instilled great confidence in me when I was young, always highlighting my predominant nose and skin. I also understood that my darker skin tone was a trait I inherited from my grandfather on my father's side. It reminded me that I was different from the rest of my family because everyone's complexion was fairer than mine. I thought that was the only thing that set me apart from them. Sadly, I was wrong.

In a world filled with racism and colorism, I never thought much about my color, no race, until I got to high school. Little did I know, I wasn't close to scratching the surface of what separated me from other people. My grandmother went from looking after me to me being placed solely in her care until she was no longer able. My parents worked during the day and sometimes at night to provide a stable roof over our heads. My brother and sister were out at school, leaving Manmie Lea and me ample time to form our precious bond. A lot of her time was dedicated to raising me.

Haiti Cherie

My parents decided I would be better situated in her arms. She raised my brother and sister, so it only seemed fitting that she would do just fine in helping to raise me. Manmie Lea and I visited Haiti on our first flight I was three years old.

We spent our time in Haiti at one of my uncle's lavish homes, which he has now turned into a resort. The beautiful seventies-styled vintage rustic Chateau' was my private playground and oasis. I remember getting lost in the endless mango, sugar cane, coconut, and guinep (Spanish lime) groves, and I'd have fresh fruit picked and juiced for breakfast and lunch. The nostalgia of my first swim in my uncle's 18-foot-deep Olympic size in-ground swimming pool will always remain with me. The collection was incredibly captivating, and despite my parent's safety concerns, I persevered in learning how to swim. They paid for private lessons for me. Certain freedom I felt when I swam brought me joy.

I was buoyant and fearless; within a year, I became a seasoned swimmer. Tiny, agile, and swift, I could glide through the pool. I admired the water almost as much as the flights my grandmama took. One of my favorite parts of our stay at my uncle's home was that he had dogs running around all over the grounds.

I adapted quickly to the culture and fell in love with the warmth of the country and its people. My six-birthday grandmother and I were in and out of Haiti as if we were on constant holiday. I became familiarized with my heritage and my mother's side of the family over the next four to five years.

I visited Haiti with my grandmother for months, never any less, until I started grade school. I absorbed many cultures during our visits, even becoming fluent in Creole, French, and Spanish. Vacations were filled with lots of joyful and warm memories. I kept my grandmother on her toes. Most memories still serve me are filled with more sensory nostalgia. The country was scorching and dry, with little to no humidity. That allowed aromatic air to flow freely when an offshore breeze. Everything from the palm trees to the spices of the food was smelt and a gust. Savory, sweet, and fresh, I enjoyed my people's cuisine and culture. Haiti has a scorching, dry climate year-round; during the winter months, it gets dewy and calm; the air is sweet in the winter. The summer months were so arid and dense. You could cut through the air with a knife.

I would beg my uncle Gerard and grandmother to spend our days by the water. I loved the ocean and the beautiful, bejeweled beaches, but my uncle's home had an Olympic-sized pool, so we didn't venture to the beach as often as I wanted. I always wondered why anyone would leave such a paradise. I can barely recollect the memories of my childhood stays in Haiti. The faces of the family seem more distant now. I can recall sounds, smells, and twilight as the sunset on the horizon. When dusk set on the island, I remember the lights from the houses on the mountaintops sparkling like diamonds, illuminating the island's night sky. I recall the nights when I would fall asleep from the long car rides home from the beach driving back to my uncle's manor in the sanctity of my grandmother's arms. My grandmother and I fostered a unique, close-knit, organic relationship filled with joy and trust with every moment we spent together. Our connection gave my parents peace of mind knowing I was in the company of someone who adored me and would raise me exceptionally well.

. When I started school, it usually continued during big breaks like summer and winter, allowing my parents time to work unapologetically. Manmie was my instant travel companion, and when we returned home from our second trip in the summer of nineteen ninety, my mother registered me for preschool. Due to the untimely placement of my birthday in November, my mother forced my way into the school system. At only three and a half years old, I became the youngest to enroll in my kindergarten class.

Also, to keep me busy, my mother enrolled me in a classical dance academy in hopes of honing my energy when I wasn't at school. Dance became my life. I instantly became a lover of technical dancing. I excelled in classical ballet, tap, and jazz. I absorbed the lessons and memorized every step. There was always something new and challenging that I wanted to master. Then teach all the other kids how to do it. At the end of every year, there was a big dance recital. My mother invested in my costume as I invested in my love of dance. I was eager to get all glammed up for recital pictures and the final curtain call.

My mother encouraged me to keep busy, and I innately fell in love with the arts. Dance was my glee, and it was in my blood. It allowed my mind and body to move collectively, teaching me focus and discipline. The day I went to the hospital, all that discipline seemed irrelevant. I lost hope to continue to strive for anything, even the ability to live. The steps couldn't land the same. I turned away from dance because it didn't serve my broken spirit or my lack of balance, and It was tough to get up from the hospital bed when I felt planted in it.

I received everything and anything a child should receive without failure except a cure. At this point in my life, I couldn't differentiate between my "picture-perfect world" and pain. I saw life changing right Infront of my eyes without even having a moment to process it all. Getting sick changed my perspective of time and my confidence. Everything wondrous became intangible and bleak. My life changed dramatically. My cognition and motor skills began to deteriorate. My existence took a back seat for about seventy-five percent of my life because of a disease. My parents were establishing what was considered the American dream when my mother had my brother and sister move to the states was possible. I believed becoming sick ruined it.

After my mother became a citizen, she sponsored Manmie Lea and my uncle Louis aka Uncle Lou Lou, my mother's youngest sibling. He was a real lady's man and didn't waste time getting acquainted. Within a year after his arrival, he had a beautiful son named Lewis. Manmie Lea tried to raise my younger cousin, and I was like two peas in a pod as he was only two years younger than me. She tried to instill in us the importance of pride in our culture, family, and manners. Young Lewis and I both were spoiled emotionally by my grandmother. My mother didn't encourage time away from work or school, and my uncle had different ideals. Though young Louis was born in the United States, his father wasn't focused enough to afford his family the same resources we had. Slowly, my uncles and wife migrated into my parent's home, and within the same year, my little sister Alisha was conceived. It was more than a whole house. It was an unpleasant time for my family dynamic as my grandmother struggled to keep the peace among her children and son-in-law. My father was up in arms with my Manmie Lea and forced my uncle and cousin to leave. They moved into an apartment across town.

Months went by, and my cousin's behavior showed no improvement. My grandmother and uncle could not keep my cousin on track due to my uncle's fight with alcoholism and my grandmother's age. Young Louis began skipping school and gave up on playing soccer, which was his sole passion. My uncle didn't like the idea of him playing a sport and how much he had to pay for Louis to be involved. Louis was a child to me. Baby cousin, yet as much I wanted to protect him, I was no match for the perplexities that would plague him nor what I was about to confront in mine.

Uncle Louis's wife became very sick after their second child, and my elderly grandmother couldn't keep young Louis from getting into trouble. She couldn't handle being a caretaker for my uncle's wife and their newborn and running after a pre-teen boy. Louis was often left to raise himself, finding a sense of family in the wrong places. My uncle fathered another child and decided to send Louis, his pregnant wife, back to Haiti as a scare tactic for Louis to straighten up. Louis arrived back in the states with a different mindset; he became resentful and disgruntled. Smoking and drinking, he stopped playing soccer and became invested and affiliated with the wrong crowd and spent years in juvenile detention, and finally ended up in prison.

My grandmother and uncle's stress resonated within the family, and it vested within me. It didn't make sense. Why couldn't we help my cousin? I was devastated, and my grandmother became overwhelmed and sad. Manmie Lea's sorrow vibrated through my family and resonated viscerally in me. When her tears began to fall, it felt like they were unending. My grandmother was an emotional person. She was remorseful, empathetic, compassionate, and generous. Though my parents couldn't give me their complete attention, Mammie Lea never neglected me, no matter how hurt she felt. Her burdens did change the dynamic of our relationship, and it was difficult to access my grandmother, but not impossible. Her energy was transcendent. She would walk across town to visit me and drop off food. She told me how she spoke to Louis and longed to see him. It hurt me because I was not in a position where I could help. If she didn't drop it off, she would occasionally have a friend deliver food to my home.

As I got sicker, my mother and grandmother's relationship became estranged, and there was nothing that could have stopped my grandmother from coming to take care of me. I needed her. However, my mother tried her best to hold it all together; my grandmother's presence always came with a need to help my cousin as his father was also grieving the news of his imprisonment. We moved, and our relationship became strained. I internalized much resentment when Manama moved out to live with my uncle. The pressure from my mother was inescapable. It took years to reconnect with my mother because of my fear of dealing with MS and her pretenses. My mother was very stern, realistic, and unapologetically by the book.

I can't recall when I saw him break down as he did when he learned I had a disease. However, she carried her entire family, finances, and my health. Her family's safety was the top priority, and the order was circumstantial. Having a two-household income in New York was necessary for two young immigrant adults and sometimes upholding three or four jobs. It was an unspoken truth that when you are old enough to work, children must contribute to the bills instead of learning how to contribute to family *wealth*. Despite how hard it was to get time off from work amidst the chaos, my mother never missed a doctor's appointment. She also made it a point to be home on her breaks to check on me, mainly if I stayed home from school, which was more often than I ever cared to do. I wouldn't see beyond that tall gate for years without accompaniment. Teenage angst and MS became my solitary confinement.

It was hard for both of my parents to conclude that they had a sick child with no diagnosis and a disease they had never heard of. It became cerebral when I was diagnosed with an ailment they had never heard of. My father never spoke about my diagnosis. My mother became my warden, and my brother became my parole officer. My siblings couldn't begin to understand my troubles, and I didn't know how to express them. Therefore, the age gap and my illness made it harder for us to bond. Their daily chores and social lives consumed them and other activities as my grief consumed me. I just progressively got sicker and became disabled while our relationships became estranged.

Multiple Sclerosis snuck up on me like a thief in the night and changed my life forever. I faced severe circumstances that I could have never imagined devastated and burdened my relationship with my family and God. Multiple Sclerosis interrupted and cut short my childhood. It forced me to grow up quickly. I had one of the most challenging times transitioning into middle school. Multiple Sclerosis stifled my social and mental growth through adolescence and adulthood. It harnessed the power to make it impossible to adjust, for half of my mind was stuck between those institutional corridors of my elementary school gymnasium and the gloomy hospital emergency room for years. I couldn't see; I was entrapped in all the pain. I had already been afflicted by such emotional, physical, and mental pain and didn't know if I could take any more. I had to fight my way back.

3

So Many questions, So Little Answers

May of 1999

"Well, do you think I'll miss my graduation and dance?" I asked my mother for the hundredth time. She never answered me, so I kept nagging her because I hated being ignored. I didn't think she could have given the immediate answer I was looking for. I scanned the bright white hospital emergency room for the nearest exit, but there was no sign. It smelled sickly and sterile in the emergency waiting room. I felt tiny, cold, and uncomfortable in such unfamiliar surroundings. The nurse called my name quickly, and my slow and lonely descent into disparity began. After my mother gave her insurance card to the billing clerk, the ER nurse was ready to see us and started a few rudimentary exams. The nurse quickly transferred me from the emergency room to a unit within an hour. The room was gloomy and dimly lit with curtains that divided the room per patient. The walls had been painted the color of eggnog left out overnight. The room had no windows for sunlight and poor ventilation. The cold, stale air kept circulating throughout the units. I could recall the noise from the construction on the grand Pavilion floor. Between the noise, anxiety, and the smell of hospital food, I became increasingly nauseous and felt a migraine creeping on. I didn't know what a migraine was, but I quickly found out. My spirit became daunted by the idea that I wouldn't leave the emergency room anytime soon, but I was still hopeful.

The confusion and time lapsing were making me irritable. Yet I couldn't do anything about it. A nurse walked and tried to focus focused on her pale hand. The hands were leathery, pasty, white, dry, and wrinkled. The nurse handed me a hospital gown. My soul dropped into the pit of my stomach, and my eyes swelled up in tears as I reached for it, annoyed. She grazed my hand while handing it off to me. Cold as they were, I grabbed it and stared at the hand with a puzzled look. The hospital gown I thought it was a bed sheet. She said my name and I shook my head from left the right and answered yes. I was confused about what to do with the gown as the nurse walked away. My mother took it from me and told me to get undressed and leave my underwear in creole. I did as instructed, and I laid back in bed with a gown on and, as requested, with the opening facing the back. I curled up and began heaving tears. My mother placed the sheet over my body and wiped the tears away, but they kept coming. The confusion continued to funnel through my mind outward to the extremities in the form of pins and needles, leaving me exhausted.

Will I ever see my friends again? Glimpses of all the new dances I learned at the fine dance academy that I would never get to share, smiles that I would never see, and time left unshared bombarded my tiny mind. My eyes searched the room for anything indicative of me leaving. I wondered why I couldn't get prescribed antibiotics and be on my merry way. The hospital shouldn't be able to hold me against my will, nor should my mother allow them to. *Who did they think they were?* I had somewhere important to be, and people were waiting for me. At an age where the simplest things become the epicenter of your life, my sixth-grade dance was what I had waited my *entire* life for. So much time passed that I wondered if my friends would even notice I was missing. All I wanted to do was get up and dance to celebrate my accomplishment of graduating from elementary school. I promised God I would do my best behavior if they allowed my parents to take me back to school.

Many questions constantly rattled through my brain, filling my mind and spirit with dark uncertainties and sadness. My time was being stolen from me. I lay there in the hospital bedroom as tiny spots began to multiply throughout my brain. At eight and a half years old, there wasn't a thought in my mind that being better behaved wouldn't get me out of the hospital, but my promises went unheard. Time stood still for me as the world kept spinning. I continued to reach out for clarity as nurses paced in and out of the unit like toy soldiers. They all marched to the same beat with the same blank expression lamenting on their faces. My mother had left me to use the restroom. I remember feeling alone and fearful. I asked several nurses several times where my mother was, and they answered with silence. Since there was no sign of my mother or a doctor, I became unnerved, and my heart was beating erratically as it sat in my belly. I began crying again for my mother like a newborn child.

It seemed as if my elementary school graduation had become my doomsday. My crowning achievement was washed out by sadness and ambiguity. I became weak, breathless, and mute. With fading hopes, I lay there against my will in that hospital bed, surrounded by dull walls and opaque gray curtains. The marching of nurses muffled the beeping from the cardiac machine attached to my chest. The chatter of the doctors grew louder outside the hospital bedroom door. I wished for their following words to be that I'm good to get back to my regular scheduled program. Their prolonging what was next on the hospital's agenda got me thinking that I may have been blindsided by the severity of what I did wrong. That's the longest I was ever left alone in a hospital since my baby sister was born. Regardless of the pain and uncertainties, I wondered how sick I was.

I cried and squealed, hoping someone would swoop in and rescue me. Neither my frustrations nor the torrential downpour of tears gave me any answers or alleviation. My antics just intensified the unearthly, foreign feelings in my flesh. It started as pins and needles, then quickly became a sensation of termites eating away at my face, arms, and legs. The more upset I became, the more vigorous the sense that The was no escaping it. The feeling became so vigorous that my face started to become numb. There was something that I had never experienced before brewing within my body, and I didn't think antibiotics would have been the answer. I went from feeling frightened to overwhelmed and disoriented within hours, mystified by the sensations I'd never experienced before; I started screaming for the doctors to let out.

I was experiencing all of what my teacher claimed she had seen. I began to brace myself for what the practitioners had to say next, even though I had already decided I wanted to leave no exceptions. I wanted to know the cause of these feelings, yet I was afraid. No one wanted to let me in on my secret. Getting up from the hospital bed was tough when I felt planted in it. The feeling of pins and needles in my legs vibrated through me and was volatile

.

I couldn't walk. As the sensations pelted me, my immune system was fighting, and my nerves were revolting; overworked and over-loaded, erupting in my body as tremors and fits were fueled by my anxiety. Although my thoughts subconsciously plagued my body, there was a little girl still hopeful and waiting for my parents and doctors to burst through the room, hand me my clothes, and tell me that I could r to school. I would even accept if they had told me that it was all a big misunderstanding and that I would be okay without any explanation. With a muddied mind, any bare minimum was acceptable if there would be any momentary relief or gain.

Nevertheless, my confusion festered throughout the walls of the hospital room. A nurse came in with more paperwork. Then she gave me the option to solicit one of my arms for my introduction to phlebotomy. I sure didn't know the reason, but before I knew it, I chose my right arm, which still is my favorite arm to get blood drawn from. I winced when she placed the "butterfly," as she called it, into the vein of my forearm. Thus began the cycle of blood work and other tests. The day was dusk, and my father and brother finally arrived at the hospital. Eager to see them both, I mustered up the energy to plaster a big, crooked smile. Our eyes instantly connected as my father walked into the hospital emergency room. He stared at me as if he didn't recognize me. My father's face began to look remote and pale. He held his head in his hands and let out a baritone sigh, then began to heave and cry. Never in my life have I witnessed a single teardrop fall from my father's eyes. Yet, there he stood, a giant crumbling, while my brother, half his size, held him tight so he wouldn't collapse.

Minutes later, my mother walked into the room, followed by the aroma of fresh New York oven-baked cheese pizza. Regal and poised as she was, I could tell she was trying to conceal her sorrow though she didn't try to make direct eye contact with me. She was holding it all together as she walked past my hospital food tray brought in by the nurse this morning, pushed it aside, and placed the pizza box near a table by my bedside. I could see she had just finished wiping tearstains away from her crimson-colored cheeks. Her pointy red nose and iris were red like the cherry tomatoes Mama Lea and I planted for the summer harvest, a dead giveaway she'd been crying.

My mother casually escorted my father and brother into the hallway. Seeing my father cry only made me further upset and confused. That pizza box only began what would ignite emotional eating habits that I would resort to suppressing my anxiety and grief. At that very moment, I reached over for the pizza box, still warm, and devoured half the pie in one sitting, and I began to fall asleep. As I was nodding off, I could hear the nurse and doctors as they stood outside in the hallway and spoke to my parents. The nurse startled me as she walked back in with a chart. She read my name out loud.

The doctor followed in alongside my parents. I jumped out of my sleep; my heart stopped and sat in my throat as the doctor read my sentence. I felt as if I knew what he would say before he spoke. I heard a loud silence, and I gasped for air. My mother asked the nurse for visitation times. My gut instincts told me it was the beginning of many questions, and I would not go home for a while. I was beside myself, unable to catch my breath. It was almost like time had stopped. It was an out-of-body experience. My body became sore as my spirit shattered, and my heart became dense. I pleaded with my mother not to leave, and she affirmed that it would be ok. Left alone that night, my mother told me she would return to tend to me in the early morning and connect the cable and phone services for my room.

I reiterated that I felt *fine* and was well enough to go home, but she exclaimed that wouldn't be happening just yet. My mother told me my older sister would visit if she couldn't make it. After they all left, I wept and sobbed heavily until I fell asleep, watching night turn into day. My sister arrived with her now ex-husband with a great breakfast from the International House of Pancakes. My worries briefly subsided because I had family and food for entertainment and comfort. That was short-lived as I began to experience more chronic symptoms after I ate a heavy breakfast. I craved my sleep, and insomnia claimed it. My sister and her husband left when I fell asleep. Mother didn't arrive until that evening with the food my grandmother had prepared for me. The food was accompanied by her signature cutlery folded between a napkin set. I ate half of the food and waited for the doctor to release me.

Hours turned into days, and my ability to comprehend my health depleted my body and weakened the chances of me being released were slim. Watching life pass me by was brutal and criminal, and I did not have anyone to save me. My worries began to consume my eight-year-old mind as nurses continued to draw blood from my veins for more tests, and even less information was given to my parents—the results of the examinations translated into inconclusive tests. Regardless of how much my mother tried to explain what was happening, I couldn't wrap my mind around what she was saying. Being young and unable to steer your mind through the cluster was a disadvantage. Older people feel less obligated to communicate effectively with the youth, or maybe they don't know how. I was kept in the darkness at one of the darkest moments in my vulnerable life. The experience hurt me in ways unimaginable. I could no longer breathe because the night was so heavy and was trying to close in on me. My angst began to sow into my chest and the pit of my belly.

One morning, I woke up to use the restroom and placed my feet on the floor. There was a lack of sensation as I tried to touch the base and realized the bed was further than I thought, or they had amputated my feet when I was sleeping. I reached over towards my feet, which were cold to the touch with no sensation. I immediately alerted the nurse. She came in, and she helped me use the restroom. Then I was quickly taken into a large white room with a large, sizeable casket-like machine. I was transferred onto the MRI bed from the gurney. I was told to lie down and place earplugs to muffle any sound and not to move. The nurse unhooked the medication from my arm and replaced it with a saline flush.

I laid back and did what I was told. The lights dimmed around me, and as soon as I closed my eyes, the machine started to rattle and tick loudly, and the earsplitting sound of the device jolted me. I moved around, looking inside the device to see if anything was broken. The sounds made it seem that something was going to explode. The tech stopped the machine and repeated that I couldn't move and that if I did not keep still, it would compromise the imaging, and the process would take even longer. He reached into a cabinet, pulled out a large piece of foam, and gently fixed it between my neck and shoulders. Then I propped my legs on a pillow. Then he asked if I was cold. I clenched my hands into a fist, trying not to move, and felt the chill in my finger-tips. Then I rubbed my arm, felt my goosebumps, and said," yes, please." The tech draped another blanket over me and asked me what music I liked. I told him to classical music, please.

My anxiety eased once the door was closed and the music came on. I thought of my dance recital that I never would attend. I felt cold and tired; within seconds, I dosed off and was interrupted by the device's loud tapping, clicking, and humming. I was in and out of sleep during the process, which lasted for three hours. Then the machine tech stopped and gave me a contrast through my IV, which would help identify and highlight any abnormalities in my brain and lumbar (vertebrate). My mother was shown my MRI (Magnetic Resonance Imaging) days after the procedure. I would try to pay attention, as she did too. I couldn't follow exactly what the doctors were saying. I hoped she did.

I remember seeing heavily populated white cloud-like structures that echoed through my MRI. He kept pointing at them and shaking his head. No one understood how these white images would affect my mental and spiritual well-being. A paranoia surged over my body. I heard my name in whispers. I can hear it clearly over the beeping of the cardiac machines and the shuffling of administration in the hallway. There was no word of when I was going home, but various mentions of tests, medication, and monitoring. Doctors placed me under a very high dosage of steroids. I concluded there was something more to why I was being held here.

My parents petitioned me to have my private room in the hospital since it would be my new residence for the summer of nineteen ninety-nine. Within a week, the porters transitioned me from the shared emergency room quarters to my space upstairs in the pediatric neurology unit. The room was large and warmer, with large bay windows that let in much natural sunlight. Flowers and balloons filled the room from family and friends that I thought had forgotten about me. Once I was there, the doctors would come in for routine examinations. I was being poked and probed like I was an exotic specimen. They hung my MRI images on a board with a light illuminating behind them, high-lighting my brain's imperfections. It was explained to my parents, and as I tried to listen in and comprehend, many abnormalities were seen. We weren't familiar with the world of neurology, nor could the doctors explain precisely why the white callous-like plaques obstructed my neu-rological pathways. Still, I felt the anomaly's cryptic tendencies. Like outdated wallpaper hung on the walls of the pediatric emergency hos-pital ward, their obsolete presence was obstructing my life. Each white spot adorned the film began weighing me physically and mentally. The lesions were eating away at my tiny mind. My conversations became vague, limited, and short. My tone was cold and lacked luster. I became so angry and exhausted that my temper became swift and intense. I thought to hell with my graduation or with dance. I just missed my grandmother, and I know she would be able to help. I never understood why she hadn't visited.

Whenever anyone asked me how I felt, I kept telling them I felt fine. That was my blanket statement. I was fine meant that I was stuck in a parallel universe that not even Dr. Strange could have gotten me out of, and I was fearful for my life. I couldn't be present in a place absorbing my youth and joy, where I desperately wanted to escape. Despite my uncomfortably, I dare not reiterate how much pain I was in because I thought it would prolong my hospital stay. It was a few weeks since I was administered, and I was physically, mentally, and emotionally exhausted. Plagued with anxiety and stress, my jaw would lock up, and body would tense, and I wouldn't be able to move. I often felt my chest tighten up, leaving me breathless as if someone had clasped their arms around my ribcage and were squeezing me for dear life. My hands became clammy, and I felt sick and nauseous whenever the hospital bedroom door opened. I refused to express this because I thought it would prolong my stay. The pain just continued to pile on.

I didn't think things could become any more confusing and complicated. I got my menstrual a month into my hospital admittance. I could hide it to save myself from further embarrassment, but quickly my mother caught on, and so did the nurses. I finally got to the bathroom and was introduced to my crooked smile (Bell's Palsy). It took a month to see what horror was happening to my body finally, but I felt its deathly prescience creeping up on me from the beginning.

4

Chronically Young and Brown

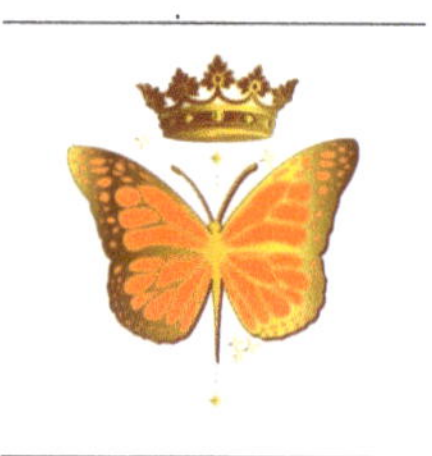

"I know why the caged bird sings"- Maya Angelou.

My days seemed as if they were on a loop. Like clockwork, doctors paced in and out, bringing other practitioners into my room for daily observations. Those that accompanied the doctor seemed young in the face as they statically walked around my hospital bed—whispering about as they looked through my charts. They vigorously wrote on their notepads as they exited my room into the hallway. They wouldn't come during visiting hours or when my mother was around.

It seemed eerie that they would only come in when I was alone.

My first account of medical negligence was when the porter took me from my room and rushed me into another room on a gurney. Not understanding what was next, I had many objections, yet I remained silent. The nurse looked me square in the eye as if she was starving her apprehensions. Yet, she proceeded to take my vital; then she gave me a tongue depressor, with instructions to place it between my teeth and bite down during the procedure if anything would hurt. Then continued to brief me on how this procedure was to help find out what was going on with me and that it shouldn't hurt much if I stayed still. With the depressor already in between my tiny teeth, I immediately tensed up and bit into the wood. The doctor walked in, followed by a few others in lab coats, and explained the procedure to all assembled in the room. "The process was to withdraw spinal fluid between the vertebrate and the spine. The sample that would be drawn would help to determine my disorder." I was already shaken and disconnected; therefore, whatever they said seemed irrelevant. I did catch him saying that the Novocain would be the worst part of the procedure, then once my back was numb, everything would go very smoothly. I knew what Novocain was because I had some stubborn baby teeth extracted at the dentist some years prior. I still couldn't wrap my mind around what was about to unveil.

I tried my best to follow directions and put on a brave face. The nurses propped me upright on the gurney under the bright hospital light and restrained me while the doctors forcefully hunched me over with the back of my hospital gown open. The anesthesiologist began the prep by sterilizing my back for the lower lumbar puncture, also known as the spinal tap. The doctor saturated the gauze and placed it on my back. As soon as I felt the cooling sensation of the anti-septic, I knew I was occupying a space that wasn't mine.

As permanent goosebumps filled my arms, so did my anxiety and the pressure to be still. I had no idea how I was supposed to feel as I wanted to stop them. I emotionally propped myself upright and braced mentally for what I thought would feel like a tooth extraction. The anesthesiologist used topical Novocain to numb the insertion area, then pushed a thin needle into my back filled with a local anesthetic to further numb around my spinal area (just a pinch, she said). I winced and bared the pain of the tiny needles. I closed my eyes and heard the loudest silence; I had visions of bright flashes of white, yellow, and blue lights strobing past as there were sealed shut.

I saw colors in the dark. I was caught in a nightmare. Tears began cascading from my eyes like a flood as I winced through the process biting as hard as I could on the tongue depressor. I heard the clanging of medical supplies, and I sat there breathless with my stomach in knots. I barely caught my breath as I tried to open my eyes; I peered through my tears and saw a long thick needle.

Another needle slid into my spine, and I screamed. I thought it was over, I tried to sit up straight, yet I was pushed down by the nurse and held hunched over and restrained by another. Then the doctors sternly told me not to move. The nurse gave me another tongue depressor, saying, "You're going to have to do your best not to move this time, honey." I took a deep breath and closed my eyes as the needle slid into my back like a hot knife through fresh ice on New Year's in New York. I kept my eyes closed again as tears continued to stream from my clenched eyelids. The needle slid in and out quicker than the first, but that didn't mean it was less painful than the first. Finally, I was asked if I was ok, and I shook my head up and down with tears from my eyes and mucus streaming from my nose. Someone handed me a tissue, and then they continued.

Another person in a lab coat took over. As the larger instrument was picked up, I heard the clanging metal sound again. At that moment, I felt helpless and grew to understand endurance and resiliency, although it would take a lifetime to master. I felt the nurses' grip tighten; I bit down so hard on the tongue decompressor that I chipped my tooth.

Violently I wailed as the extraction began and ended untunefully. The *acting physician* stepped aside as he apologized to his colleagues. Another white coat stepped in. I felt unnerved because it was probably a pre-med student who didn't pass their finals and got stuck in summer school. Yet uninterrupted, the next student drove a needle into my spine. I cried and screamed, begged for mercy, and suddenly, I heard knocking at the door and my mother's voice on the other side. My entire body was shaking because I was in intense and blinding pain.

Finally, my mother forced her way into the room and demanded to know what was happening. The licensed physician took over and administered the rest of the procedure. When the syringe connected to my spine again, I felt a rush of fire followed by extraction of cool being pulled from my body. The spinal tap incident entirely shaped my perspective of pain. It was as if my youth was being extracted from my soul. My mother often spoke about the pre-med students even being in the room that day and why she wasn't told about the procedure. She didn't comprehend why no one intervened. I didn't know why I couldn't tell them not to touch me. My fear overshadowed any assertiveness that existed. I was silenced without a word; I began crumbling without comprehension. I was frozen in time.

I was exhausted and became extraordinarily withdrawn and melancholy; I flew into a great depression. My spirit was numb, and my vulnerability was blatant and superficial. This pain was more than a scraped knee; it was a sickness peeling off layers of my adolescence like paint on an old windowpane. The pain was considerable and stayed with me throughout my early adult life. My spinal tap left me hypersensitive in my lower back, which would last me a lifetime—it was the beginning of an out-of-body experience. I couldn't believe this series of events that were happening to me.

After the procedure, the nurse placed a thick piece of gauze where the syringes entered. I was moved back into my room, cried, and laid on my side amidst the darkness. With cold fresh sterile white linen sheets draped over my tiny frame, I lay there miserable, with my mind in a fog. My wounds remained open for quite some time, constantly oozing fluid. It made it even harder to get out of bed, yet that didn't stop me from trying, especially when soiled sheets were involved. I tried earnestly to get up and use the bathroom, but I feared everyone would see my Tuesday underwear when it was Saturday. The pain in my back was vicious, and I didn't know if the procedure kept me from being mobile or was it the sickness. I was too weak to walk, stand, shower, or go alone to use the bathroom. It was painful deciding if I should hold my bladder or risk walking to the bathroom because I couldn't just pee on myself, then I'd be a baby. I no longer wanted to move nor associate with others of the sense of sheer embarrassment. I was in extreme agony and confusion. All my cries were useless, and all my questions were going unanswered. I grew angry and presumed that I didn't matter.

The millions of fire ants marching up and down my body constantly ravaged my legs, face, and arms. No one knew because no one would give me a chance to convey my feelings, nor did I understand how to. As fast as doctors came in and saw me, they left quickly. The sensation was so vigorous at times that it caused my whole right side to go numb and I ultimately became paralyzed for moments. Those few moments felt like hours of agony. I began to consider what if I never walked out of the hospital the way I walked in; mentally, physically, emotionally, or spiritually. I laid there, day after day, and wondered what was in the IV and steroid drip. I was paralyzed by pain, fear, and worry. I was wishing and wondering when all this agony would stop.

On one occasion, while my bathroom was being cleaned, the nurse assisted me in using the guest restroom a few doors down from mine. It had to be the most excellent room in the pediatric ward because it was adorned with all the Disney princesses on the walls. It had perfect lighting and large vanity with a mirror to my left. I dragged myself into the restroom with the nurse's aide and locked the door behind me. I tried to use the bathroom but quickly realized it was impossible to move without assistance, so I held on to the sink. I looked at my reflection in the mirror, and I was repulsed. The Bel's Palsy took over my entire right side. I stared at my review for what seemed to be hours —widening and closing my eyes, scrutinizing its imperfections. *What's happening with me? How am I supposed to go to school like this?* I wondered as I stared at my reflection and cried. The nurse knocked on the door, and I told her I'd be right out. I used the restroom, held on to the handrails and skink to stand up, and washed my hands and face.

During my next few weeks in the hospital, the numbing sensation began funneling through my face, lips, nose, and eyes. Even my scalp was without feeling. It was as if a fuzzy thin film was laid over my face, almost like a spider web. I tried to wipe it away, wash it out, cry it and even sleep it away. Nothing worked. I was battling intense vertigo every time I lifted my torso. Disoriented and dizzy, I was scared and bewildered as my migraines persisted. Is this what a hangover felt like? The pain taunted me. *"Was my brain crowning through my skull?"* because I thought my head would split open. The pounding forced me to sleep, and, as I expressed to the doctor, I was told it was normal.

At night I would hear and feel the constant fluttering in my ear. It was as if little moths were flapping their wings in my canal, and their *larvae were probably eating at my brain*. My imagination ran wild as I tried to make sense of what was happening to me internally. The flutter coincided with the facial numbness. I also had constant tremors, which surged through my spine from my fingertips, and ran up to my lips. The pain, alongside the earthquakes, made it very hard to concentrate and even caused me a loss of appetite. Not even my grandmother's food could stir up my desire. During the day, my eyes were always dreary and tired no matter how long I slept, for I no longer had a typical sleep pattern. My fatigue was relentless. I could fall asleep anywhere at any time. I would get very restless at night and try to get out of bed. The doctors and nurses urged me to stay in bed, but my mind wanted my body to escape. When I had the urge and found some strength, I would focus enough energy to get out of bed and roam the white hollow hallways late in the evening or at night when it was quiet, desolate, and no one was around. I didn't know where I thought I was going, with the IV drip dragging behind me like a lost puppy. I hung on to the blue ceramic railing that lined the hallway, and carts filled with medical supplies to keep me from falling until a nurse walked by and escorted me back to my room.

I became a fragmented existential version of myself. I felt mangled, confused, and exhausted when I was back in bed. I tried to break free almost every other night, but with no plan and immense pain, I didn't have anywhere to escape. Like angels, the nurses were always there to apprehend me whenever I found courage. On one occasion, the doctor came in for an examination. I felt better in my spirit like it was time to *show him*. Regardless of conflicting thoughts, I told the doctor I felt well. He looked at me, and I got out of bed. "*I can tap dance; just watch!*" I went right into a dance step that I remembered from my tap recital, which I never had the chance to attend. I shuffled my right foot and took one step to the left, and never landed back on my right foot. I was so embarrassed that I wanted to crawl out of my skin. If it weren't for him standing by, I would have fallen on my face and taken everything attached to me down with me. The nurses would lecture me about my safety. I didn't want to hear a word and didn't care. Everything seemed distant, and my energy level declined as I became emotionally desensitized. My vibrant confidence began to recoil and cower. My ego was as fragile as the mess that was in my mind. I was in a sunken place. My thoughts became grimaced and gray.

The nurses would bring video game councils and play at my bedside to raise my spirits. I wasn't interested in any social interaction. Trying to be kind, I never turned down a game. I painfully squinted and smiled, wanting to refocus my eyes on the television screen and the buttons on the remote control. I displayed sore grins during my Nintendo 64 and Sony PlayStation rematch games. My attitude kept people at arm's length and kept them from asking me am I okay a million times. God knew that once was more than enough for me. My conversations were short and careless, and my tone was cold and lacked luster. I didn't want to play games with the nurses, but I did pass some time because there was nothing I could do.

I grew tired so quickly, and soon, they would leave. I often was left alone and thought to hell with my graduation or dance. I just missed my grandmother and wondered why she hadn't visited. Was it because I stopped eating the food she sent for me? I had a loss of appetite. The perplexity of what was happening to me angered me to the point where visitors, flowers, and their good wishes became a bore, inconvenience, and a bother. I was embarrassed and frustrated, and I tried to play sleep to evade the question, *"how are you feeling?"* I knew My answer made no difference anyhow.

As if matters couldn't get any worse, my first menstrual cycle appeared in the hospital that summer. I didn't know quite what to make of it; I was overwhelmed and ashamed. I hid it for a time by wrapping my underwear with paper tissue for the first day or two until my mother noticed and found residual blood. She brought me my first panty liner because my cycle was very light. It disappeared within three days. It was a very odd time for my period to make its grand entry.

During my last days at the hospital, I could barely see without placing immense strain on my eyes. I wasn't stable enough to play video games. My vision was unclear, murky, and daunting, both literally and figuratively. My eyesight became blurry and doubled at times (diplopia) and ran its course vehemently. I suffered from involuntary rapid eye movement; optic neuritis, and I thought I would go blind. The double vision made it hard for me to concentrate and walk. My balance only worsened in time, but my vision improved months later. The headaches were constant. The facial paralysis intensified to the point where I would drool out the side of my mouth without feeling a thing. The lack of sensation made me manic and depressed. I was losing all my senses and further losing touch with reality.

Everything, especially my future, seemed so unclear. My aspirations and dreams became farfetched and faded. I lost the luster of what it meant to be a child. My smile became obsolete. As the summer ended, I experienced disturbing emotions and pain, making me quick-tempered and more aggressive. Happiness became a foreign emotion for me. The spark I once held in my soul began to disappear and extinguish. I felt heavy and sluggish throughout the day, yet I couldn't sleep as much as I searched for it at night. My new life was adorned with shades of gray and black, the highlights of my solitude. The innocence in my eyes began to look austere. I was caught in a void, unable to express myself or tame my emotions. I began to feel safer alone.

The day I was discharged, I left a different version of myself than when I went in. It was tough for me to walk or do anything alone. Mammie Lea came with my change of clothing and an abundance of calm during my discharge and helped me get dressed. I had limited mobility and a lack of awareness of my body's capabilities. I was wheeled out, and my father helped me into my mom's BMW X5, which was inconvenient for me to get in and out of because it was a truck, and my legs felt extremely heavy. It was exhausting to lift them. Under doctor's orders, I was sent home to quarantine for the final days of summer. The state of quarantine seemed to last a lot longer than intended, and when I first came home, it was my choice. I never returned to my elementary school to pick up my diploma nor visited any friends.

Vulnerability

I refused to show any weakness or pain in public. I didn't want anyone to ask me how I felt because *"okay"* was my go-to answer. There wasn't anything anyone could do. I became more tolerant of my pain and a great fabricator of my circumstances. I became stubborn, defiant, and angry. In my pubescent stage, it was solidified that the thought of me showing any sign of fragility made me more of a child, and no one would take me seriously. I concluded that I had to choose a stance either; be a child and show my hurt and pain or buck up and put my big girl pants on. Maybe if I had stood up for myself on that day of my hospital admittance and ran away, I would have been better off. I often blamed myself. I assumed it was my fault for letting the doctors tell me what to do. Through my broken and crooked smiles, I became an expert in hiding my pain. I began to build a tolerance for pain instead of showing signs of vulnerability regardless of how internally my body felt.

My seemingly never-ending nightmare kept my eyes overflowing with tears and sorrow. They would dry up and leave remnants of salt stains that would flood over again. My grandmother would cry at times, cried with me, wiping my tears as hers fell. I hated to see her upset.

Upon my arrival home, I was greeted by tons of mail and a whole house. The first letter received was a large envelope that sealed my diploma, which I didn't think I deserved. The rest of the mail was from my new school, congratulating me on my acceptance and what was required of me. In one of the larger, heavier envelopes were my schedule, a list of textbooks, and a summer reading list. I didn't know how to deal with being sick in junior high school, but I had to figure it out. Unfortunately, I only had days until summer was over, although that didn't stop my mother and brother from reassuring me that my summer homework would be done and handed in on time. I was in such distress.

My days seemed as if they were on a loop. Like clockwork, doctors paced in and out, bringing other practitioners into my room for daily observations. Those that accompanied the doctor seemed young in the face as they statically walked around my hospital bed—whispering about as they looked through my charts and vigorously writing on their notepads as they exited my room into the hallway. They wouldn't come during visiting hours or when my mother was around.

It seemed eerie that they would only come in when I was alone. My first account of medical negligence was when the porter took me from my room and rushed me into another room on a gurney. Not understanding what was next, I had many objections, yet I remained silent. The nurse looked me square in the eye as if she had some appre-hensions. Yet, she proceeded to take my blood pressure and temperature. Then she gave me a tongue depressor, with instructions to place it between my teeth and bite down during the procedure if anything would hurt. Then continued to brief me on how this procedure was to help find out what was going on with me and that it shouldn't hurt much if I stayed still. With the depressor already in between my tiny teeth, I immediately tensed up and bit into the wood. The doctor walked in, followed by a few others in lab coats, and explained the procedure to all assembled in the room. "The process was to withdraw spinal fluid between the vertebrate and the spine. The sample that would be drawn would help to determine my disorder." I was already shaken and dis-connected; therefore, whatever they said seemed irrelevant. I did catch him saying that the Novocain would be the worst part of the procedure, then once my back was numb, everything would go very smoothly. I knew what Novocain was because I had some stubborn baby teeth extracted at the dentist some years prior. I still couldn't wrap my mind around what was about to unveil.

I tried my best to follow directions and put on a brave face. The nurses propped me upright on the gurney under the bright hospital light and restrained me while the doctors forcefully hunched me over with the back of my hospital gown open. The anesthesiologist began the prep by sterilizing my back for the lower lumbar puncture, also known as the Spinal Tap. The doctor saturated the gauze and placed it on my back. As soon as I felt the cooling sensation of the anti-septic, I knew I was occupying a space that wasn't mine.

As permanent goosebumps filled my arms, so did my anxiety and the pressure to be still. I had no idea how I was supposed to feel as I wanted to stop them, but I froze. I emotionally propped myself upright and braced mentally for what I thought would feel like a tooth extraction. The anesthesiologist used topical Novocain to numb the insertion area, then pushed a thin needle into my back filled with a local anesthetic to further numb around my spinal area (just a pinch, she said). I winced and bared the pain of the tiny needles. I closed my eyes as I heard the loudest silence; I had visions of bright flashes of white, yellow, and blue strobing past my inner eyelids.

I saw colors in the dark. I thought this must be a nightmare. Tears began cascading from my eyes like a flood as I winced through the process biting as hard as I could on the tongue depressor. I heard the clanging of medical supplies, and I sat there breathless with my stomach in knots. I barely caught my breath as I tried to open my eyes; I peered through my tears and saw a long thick needle.

Another needle slid into my spine, and I screamed. I thought it was over, I tried to sit up straight, yet I was pushed down by the nurse and held hunched over and restrained by another. Then the doctors sternly told me not to move. The nurse gave me another tongue depressor, saying, "You're going to have to do your best not to move this time, honey." I took a deep breath and closed my eyes as the needle slid into my back like a hot knife through fresh ice on New Year's in New York. I kept my eyes closed again as tears continued to stream from my clenched eyelids. The needle slid in and out quicker than the first, but that didn't mean it was less painful than the first. Finally, I was asked if I was ok, and I shook my head up and down with tears from my eyes and mucus streaming from my nose. Someone handed me a tissue, and then they continued.

Another person in a lab coat took over. As the larger instrument was picked up, I heard the clanging metal sound again. At that moment, I felt helpless and grew to understand endurance and resiliency, although it would take a lifetime to master. I felt the nurses' grip tighten; I bit down so hard on the tongue decompressor that I chipped my tooth.

Violently I wailed as the extraction began and ended untunefully. The *acting physician* stepped aside as he apologized to his colleagues. Another white coat stepped in. I felt unnerved because it was probably a pre-med student who didn't pass their finals and got stuck in summer school. Yet uninterrupted, the next student drove a needle into my spine. I cried and screamed, begged for mercy, and suddenly, I heard knocking at the door and my mother's voice on the other side. My entire body was in intense, blinding pain and shaking.

Finally, my mother forced her way into the room and demanded to know what was happening. The licensed physician took over and administered the rest of the procedure. When the syringe connected to my spine again, I felt a rush of fire followed by extraction of cool being pulled from my body. The spinal tap incident entirely shaped my perspective of pain. It was as if my youth was being extracted from my soul. My mother often spoke about the pre-med students even being in the room that day and why she wasn't told about the procedure. She didn't comprehend why no one intervened. I didn't know why I couldn't tell them not to touch me. My fear overshadowed any assertiveness that existed. I was silenced without a word; I began crumbling without comprehension.

I was exhausted and became extraordinarily withdrawn and melancholy; I flew into a great depression. My spirit was numb, and my vulnerability was blatant and superficial. This pain was more than a scraped knee; it was a sickness peeling off layers of my adolescence like paint on an old windowpane. The pain was considerable and stayed with me throughout my early adult life. My spinal tap left me hypersensitive in my lower back, which would last me a lifetime—it was the beginning of an out-of-body experience. I couldn't believe this series of events that were happening to me.

After the procedure, the nurse placed a thick piece of gauze where the syringes entered. I was moved back into my room, cried, and laid on my side amidst the darkness. With cold fresh sterile white linen sheets draped over my tiny frame, I lay there miserable, with my mind in a fog. My wounds remained open for quite some time, constantly oozing fluid. It made it even harder to get out of bed, yet that didn't stop me from trying, especially when soiled sheets were involved. I tried earnestly to get up and use the bathroom, but I feared everyone would see my Tuesday underwear when it was Saturday. The pain in my back was vicious, and I didn't know if the procedure kept me from being mobile or was it the sickness. I was too weak to walk, stand, shower, or go alone to use the bathroom. It was painful deciding if I should hold my bladder or risk walking to the bathroom because I couldn't just pee on myself, then I'd be a baby. I no longer wanted to move nor associate with others of the sense of sheer embarrassment. I was in extreme agony and confusion. All my cries were useless, and all my questions were going unanswered. I grew angry and presumed that I didn't matter.

The millions of fire ants marching up and down my body constantly ravaged my legs, face, and arms. No one knew because no one would give me a chance to convey my feelings, nor did I understand how to. As fast as doctors came in and saw me, they left quickly. The sensation was so vigorous at times that it caused my whole right side to go numb and I ultimately became paralyzed for moments. Those few moments felt like hours of agony. I began to consider what if I never walked out of the hospital the way I walked in; mentally, physically, emotionally, or spiritually. I laid there, day after day, and wondered what was in the IV and steroid drip. I was paralyzed by pain, fear, and worry. I was wishing and wondering when all this agony would stop.

On one occasion, while my bathroom was being cleaned, the nurse assisted me in using the guest restroom a few doors down from mine. It had to be the most excellent room in the pediatric ward because it was adorned with all the Disney princesses on the walls. It had perfect lighting and large vanity with a mirror to my left. I dragged myself into the restroom with the nurse's aide and locked the door behind me. I tried to use the bathroom but quickly realized it was impossible to move without assistance, so I held on to the sink. I looked at my reflection in the mirror, and I was repulsed. The Bel's Palsy took over my entire right side. I stared at my review for what seemed to be hours —widening and closing my eyes, scrutinizing its imperfections. *What's happening with me? How am I supposed to go to school like this?* I wondered as I stared at my reflection and cried. The nurse knocked on the door, and I told her I'd be right out. I used the restroom, held on to the handrails and skink to stand up, and washed my hands and face.

During my next few weeks in the hospital, the numbing sensation began funneling through my face, lips, nose, and eyes. Even my scalp was without feeling. It was as if a fuzzy thin film was laid over my face, almost like a spider web. I tried to wipe it away, wash it out, cry it and even sleep it away. Nothing worked. I was battling intense vertigo every time I lifted my torso. Disoriented and dizzy, I was scared and bewildered as my migraines persisted. Is this what a hangover felt like? The pain taunted me. "*Was my brain crowning through my skull?*" because I thought my head would split open. The pounding forced me to sleep, and, as I expressed to the doctor, I was told it was normal.

At night I would hear and feel the constant fluttering in my ear. It was as if little moths were flapping their wings in my canal, and their *larvae were probably eating at my brain*. My imagination ran wild as I tried to make sense of what was happening to me internally. The flutter coincided with the facial numbness. I also had constant tremors, which surged through my spine from my fingertips, and ran up to my lips. The pain, alongside the earthquakes, made it very hard to concentrate and even caused me a loss of appetite. Not even my grandmother's food could stir up my desire. During the day, my eyes were always dreary and tired no matter how long I slept, for I no longer had a sleep pattern. My fatigue was relentless. I could fall asleep anywhere at any time. I would get very restless at night and try to get out of bed. The doctors and nurses urged me to stay in bed, but my mind wanted my body to escape. When I had the urge and found some strength, I would focus enough energy to get out of bed and roam the white hollow hallways late in the evening or at night when it was quiet, desolate, and no one was around. I didn't know where I thought I was going, with the IV drip dragging behind me like a lost puppy. I hung on to the blue ceramic railing that lined the hallway, and carts filled with medical supplies to keep me from falling until a nurse walked by and escorted me back to my room.

I became a fragmented existential version of myself. I felt mangled, confused, and exhausted when I was back in bed. I tried to break free almost every other night, but with no plan and immense pain, I didn't have anywhere to escape. Like angels, the nurses were always there to apprehend me whenever I found courage. On one occasion, the doctor came in for an examination. I felt better in my spirit like it was time to *show him*. Regardless of conflicting thoughts, I told the doctor I felt well. He looked at me, and I got out of bed. *"I can tap dance; just watch!"* I went right into a dance step that I remembered from my tap recital, which I never had the chance to attend. I shuffled my right foot and took one step to the left, and never landed back on my right foot. I was so embarrassed that I wanted to crawl out of my skin. If it weren't for him standing by, I would have fallen on my face and taken everything attached to me down with me. The nurses would lecture me about my safety. I didn't want to hear a word and didn't care. Everything seemed distant, and my energy level declined as I became emotionally desensitized. My vibrant confidence began to recoil and cower. My ego was as fragile as the mess that was in my mind. I was in a sunken place. My thoughts became grimaced and gray.

The nurses would bring video game councils and play at my bedside to raise my spirits. I wasn't interested in any social interaction. Trying to be kind, I never turned down a game. I painfully squinted and smiled, wanting to refocus my eyes on the television screen and the buttons on the remote control. I displayed sore grins during my Nintendo 64 and Sony PlayStation rematch games. My attitude kept people at arm's length and kept them from asking me am I okay a million times. God knew that once was more than enough for me. My conversations were short and careless, and my tone was cold and lacked luster. I didn't want to play games with the nurses, but I did pass some time because there was nothing I could do.

I grew tired so quickly, and soon, they would leave. I often was left alone and thought to hell with my graduation or dance. I just missed my grandmother and wondered why she hadn't visited. Was it because I stopped eating the food she sent for me? I had a loss of appetite. The perplexity of what was happening to me angered me to the point where visitors, flowers, and their good wishes became a bore, inconvenience, and a bother. I was embarrassed and frustrated, and I tried to play sleep to evade the question, *"how are you feeling?"* I knew My answer made no difference anyhow.

As if matters couldn't get any worse, my first menstrual cycle appeared in the hospital that summer. I didn't know quite what to make of it; I was overwhelmed and ashamed. I hid it for a time by wrapping my underwear with paper tissue for the first day or two until my mother noticed and found residual blood. She brought me my first panty liner because my cycle was very light. It disappeared within three days. It was a very odd time for my period to make its grand entry.

During my last days at the hospital, I could barely see without placing immense strain on my eyes. I wasn't stable enough to play video games. My vision was unclear, murky, and daunting, both literally and figuratively. My eyesight became blurry and doubled at times (diplopia) and ran its course vehemently. I suffered from involuntary rapid eye movement; optic neuritis, and I thought I would go blind. The double vision made it hard for me to concentrate and walk. My balance only worsened in time, but my vision improved months later. The headaches were constant. The facial paralysis intensified to the point where I would drool out the side of my mouth without feeling a thing. The lack of sensation made me manic and depressed. I was losing all my senses and further losing touch with reality.

Everything, especially my future, seemed so unclear. My aspirations and dreams became farfetched and faded. I lost the luster of what it meant to be a child. My smile became obsolete. As the summer ended, I experienced disturbing emotions and pain, making me quick-tempered and more aggressive. Happiness became a foreign emotion for me. The spark I once held in my soul began to disappear and extinguish. I felt heavy and sluggish throughout the day, yet I couldn't sleep as much as I searched for it at night. My new life was adorned with shades of gray and black, the highlights of my solitude. The innocence in my eyes began to look austere. I was caught in a void, unable to express myself or tame my emotions. I began to feel safer alone.

The day I was discharged, I left a different version of myself than when I went in. It was tough for me to walk or do anything alone. Mammie Lea came with my change of clothing and an abundance of calm during my discharge and helped me get dressed. I had limited mobility and a lack of awareness of my body's capabilities. I was wheeled out, and my father helped me into my mom's BMW X5. Under doctor's orders, I was sent home to quarantine for the final days of summer. The state of quarantine seemed to last a lot longer than intended, and when I first came home, it was my choice. I never returned to my elementary school to pick up my diploma nor visited any friends.

Vulnerability

I refused to show any weakness or pain in public. I didn't want anyone to ask me how I felt because *"okay"* was my go-to answer. There wasn't anything anyone could do. I became more tolerant of my pain and a great fabricator of my circumstances. I became stubborn, defiant, and angry. In my pubescent stage, it was solidified that the thought of me showing any sign of fragility made me more of a child, and no one would take me seriously. I concluded that I had to choose a stance either; be a child and show my hurt and pain or buck up and put my big girl pants on. Maybe if I had stood up for myself on that day of my hospital admittance and ran away, I would have been better off as I often blamed myself. I assumed it was my fault for letting the doctors tell me what to do. Through my broken and crooked smiles, I became an expert in hiding my pain. I began to build a tolerance for pain instead of showing signs of vulnerability regardless of how internally my body felt.

My seemingly never-ending nightmare kept my eyes overflowing with tears and sorrow. They would dry up and leave remnants of salt stains that would flood again. My grandmother, of times, cried with me, and when I hated to see her upset.

Upon my arrival home, I was greeted by tons of mail and a whole house. The first letter received was a large envelope that sealed my diploma, which I didn't think I deserved. The rest of the mail was from my new school, congratulating me on my acceptance and what was required of me. In one of the larger, heavier envelopes were my schedule, a list of textbooks, and a summer reading list. I didn't know how to deal with being sick in junior high school, but I had to figure it out. Unfortunately, I only had days until summer was over, although that didn't stop my mother and brother from reassuring me that my summer homework would be done and handed in on time. I was in such distress.

5

Decomposition of My Tiny Spotted Mind

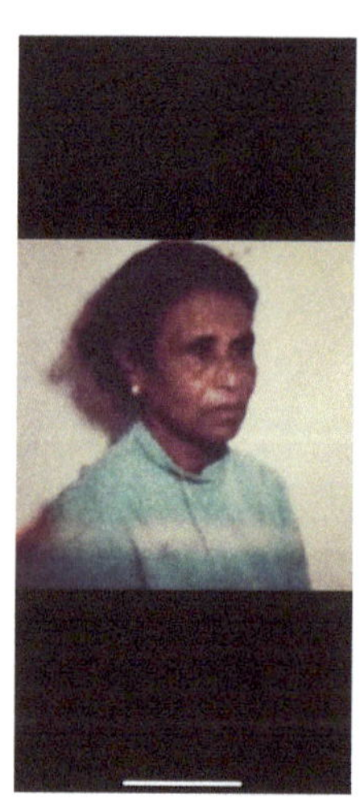

Manmie Lea

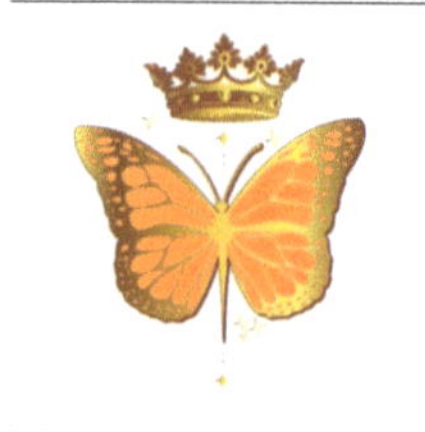

"There is no greater agony than bearing an untold story inside of you"-
Mya Angelou.

August 1999

August 1999

As dusk set on my days, so did the sun on my health. An unknown disease began to run its course two years before my diagnosis in 2001. My symptoms cast a web of hurt and darkness, hovering over my entire body and lively hood. MS made it hard for me to get a grip on reality. I wept tirelessly that summer and the next twenty years that followed. As time changed, so did my reasons why I could no longer spend my time on earth in this type of pain.

I used to bask in the sunlight as a child; I then began to find comfort in the vastness of the darkness. Spending lonely nights in the pediatric ward of the hospital started my normalization of me finding comfort in darkness and isolation. The quiet and gloom of the hospital allowed me to find reassurance to slowly let go and yet quickly accept whatever I was being told in hopes that whoever knew the answer on how to stop my pain would come to my rescue. When I finally got discharged, I found comfort in my bedroom but not in my home. Visibly my health declined rapidly and silently during the months after leaving the hospital with little hope. Members of my family and friends continued to visit me, gilded with plastered smiles, trying not to hurt my fragile ego. They wanted to sell me tall tales of how well I looked and hoped I would get well soon. Little did they know that soon wasn't in my future. They couldn't begin to comprehend the torture I felt inside, so I smiled in agreement. I didn't believe in anything anymore because I couldn't grasp what was happening. I didn't understand where this pain came from and why God would forsake me. I couldn't figure out how to get around or get past it.

While in my darkest hours, I pondered questions like, *Does God exist? Who or what Manmie Lea and I were praying to? And what did I do so wrong the warrant this mistreatment? What can I do to fix it?* My mind, body, and spirit searched for these explanations for over a decade and a half.

Even though I was finally home, I felt like I was just a guest in my house. I would lay in the darkness in pain, wishing that all of *it* would go away. I was having terrible migraines, mood swings, and nausea. I felt mystified and numb with pain. The agony wouldn't allow me to have an appetite. Manmie Lea couldn't rest knowing that I wasn't eating. As I lay still in my room, I would hear the wooden stairs begin to the creek. The familiar scent of lavender, amber, and mint permeated the hallway into my room. She was the perfect calm to my storm. The truce would only come around when Manmie Lea came to hold me; her warm embrace banished it all. She went up the stairs with freshly brewed tea and helped me drink it. My belly was often full of the tea grandmother had newly brewed from the garden. Straight off the stove, she would blow the steam off the top, warning me that it was hot and needed to be drunk as warm as possible. Holding the mug's handle and bottom with a napkin, I would also blow on the tea. I would tell her it was too hot then Manami Lea placed it by my bedside. A large nutmeg ball was on the same plate which held the teacup. While she went back downstairs to cook, I was instructed to finish the tea and place a nutmeg ball in my mouth.

I did what I was told to, but I didn't give what she said any merit. Not because I didn't believe it but because the nerve pain and facial muscle dysmorphia hadn't instantaneously gone away. Both nutmeg and tea were full of anti-inflammatory healing properties and helped soothe my symptoms and increase blood circulation. Still, my inconsistency wouldn't allow me to alleviate my pains. Sometimes she would lie beside me as I fell asleep. I tried to sleep as much as possible before the pain and muscle spasms interrupted me. When I woke up, grandma quickly got a warm washcloth infused with salt on my forehead. I also learned that anti-inflammatory properties like magnesium, zinc, iron, and potassium are found in saltwater, helping to reduce my temperature and alleviate the pressure from migraines. My migraines began a week after the spinal tap. They were long, agonizing, and excruciating and stopped my appetite.

She would then hold me close and rock me while she hummed and sang me a French lullaby: *"Lavi passe com un reive"*, translated to "Life passes by like a dream." I fell asleep to her heartbeat peacefully. Her essence was like voodoo to my soul. It placed me in a trance that soothed me into a still, almost supernatural calm state. Asleep, I would lay asleep as she softly patted my backside and sang to me like a new-born baby.

Moments passed, and like clockwork, the migraines began to pierce through my brain; they would wake me back up. The fatigue dragged my soul. All the screaming, pantomiming, and flaring of my arms, contorting my body, consistent sleepless nights, and crying for days, exhausted me. I thought the madness wouldn't end. It felt like my brain was splitting through my skull. Only she made everything stand still when so much chaos was happening within my mind and body.

Facial drooping and numbness made it much less enjoyable for me to eat; the numbness hindered my taste buds. My grandmother was torn between feeling bad for me and doing her best to try to help me cope. These episodes would go on anywhere from minutes to hours at a time. When these chronic episodes would happen, I'd be out of com-mission for days. MS caused me to feel inadequate from day one. It felt cerebral, especially when school began. I didn't think it was possible that I would ever catch up or be welcomed by other students. I would only be so reluctant to receive support from my classmates. The fear of failure consumed me, and classes had just begun. I wanted to slip away in my sleep. Maybe God would absolve my parents' most significant burden. I needed to be the least of anyone's worries. I believed I was a burden not only on myself but on everyone I met. Regardless of how I felt, Manmie Lea always held me close and never was from me, and my mother was not too far from her.

During the day, I tried to sleep away my pain at all costs. My most significant fear was confronting it. In my slumber, I was numb for a time. When I would open my eyes only to feel the haunting pain again in my brain and limbs, it felt as if the pressure leaned against the vertebrate and forefront of my skull and temporal lobes. The darkness was never mine to claim, but it became my comfort until the pain found me again.

Falling into the deep

As the summer ended, my mother spoke of where I was to take the bus and how she would do her best to drop me off every morning before she went to work. She also mentioned that I could catch a ride with one of my next-door neighbors, whose children attended the same school. The children were in Latin School, the middle school covering grades six through eight. We learned and studied Latin for three years and wore maroon-colored blazers during those years. I didn't wrap my mind around the fact that the children all had begun their high school education in the sixth grade; I was walking into a year's worth of knowledge and relationships already being fostered. Therefore, coming into as a seventh grader, I arrived reclused by no fault of my own nor the students, but I was a child with sickness with no cure. I felt like the elephant in the room.

I became thirsty, looking for someone to talk to that would understand me because I didn't understand. I craved a sense of belonging. I didn't see myself when I looked at the pamphlets, nor did I see myself in those school hallways... How could anyone understand? I kept my disease a secret as much as I could. Once I didn't feel an exchange of energy from the children from my new school, I began brandishing myself as a vigilante and building a fortress sealed with an unflinching eerie static calm. I sought asylum from the public for years. No emotional or physical pain, twitching, slurred speech, the embarrassment of stumbling, tripping over and falling short, or missed opportunities could have been noted if I had stayed alone. Just me and my secret. In the darkness, no one knew, no one could see me; in the dark, no one could judge me, and disease was beneath me.

6

The Tragedy

"A sore smile can hide a million tears and a lifetime of sorrow." Diana Lea Maisonneuve"

What I thought to be the end of my world became the beginning of my life's most considerable growing pain. Multiple Sclerosis opened a new world of adventures, filled with obstacles saturated with trials, tribulations, tragedy, tears, and triumphs.

I no longer grieve for the child I lost to P.O.M.S (Pediatric Onset Multiple Sclerosis). I put *her* away in a safe place, my ever-beating heart. I vigilantly protect *her* from anything that doesn't allow *her* the freedom to be all *she can* be. I ward away all pain, harm, and confusion of any kind. When she cries, I wipe her tears and give her reassurance.

As an adolescent, I was disturbed and haunted by the pain and uncertainty of my future. Now, I'm humbled by the memories that echoed in my nightmares. I dread to revisit what I have already experienced and repeat the battles I've already fought. I cannot regress to the days decked with ambiguity and fear. Multiple sclerosis is the epidemy of ambiguity, slighted my better judgment and fractured my mental state. Multiple Sclerosis stripped me of my childhood beyond what therapy could ever repair, though I wasn't reluctant enough to be given any. I wasn't equipped with the tools to get to the other side of this mountain. I needed to figure out what I needed, deserved then wanted. I was too young to conclude to those standards. Learning to attain that knowledge would take substantial time, patience, and the acquisition of awareness. As soon as the doctor read my diagnosis aloud to my parents and me, my heart began to race, and my clock began to tik. I ran to beat it in every wrong way possible. Because of my experiences, I learned to put up a fight and get up with every knockout and fix my crown. I never thought I had any other choice.

Every doctor's appointment was a constant reminder that my life was becoming shackled to a monster - enslaved and bullied. My spirit became shattered. Now and then, I stumbled on a missing piece to my infinite and intricate puzzle. Multiple Sclerosis's ever-changing symptoms consistently had me resetting my mind and body to endure the battle with a mysterious anomalous glitch that could not be solved. I had to come to terms with that.

There was a time when I thought wearing my older sister's ill-fitting polyester shirt to school and not getting caught was cool. I thirsted for regular school activities, chores, and social events like birthday parties, girl scouts, and dance lessons. Multiple Sclerosis had cast a shade over all that made gave me joy. My perfect bubble was ruptured, and my whole world imploded on me. All my challenges made me feel like I was running through quicksand, literally and figuratively. I became trapped in a foreign body. I lost control of my body, and my mind was clinching to my soul for salvation. These changes and challenges dragged me mentally, physically, and emotionally day in and day out. I barely recognized myself. Before my eleventh birthday, I was vindicated of normalcy, and my disease obstructed my daily childhood routines and existence. Everything came to a standstill as I approached the closing of one chapter and the beginning of the next.

I would have never suspected that I would face or even get

through such adversities. When I was first admitted to the hospital, my mother constantly reminded me to stay strong, not that I had strength, but because she wanted me to build my resilience authentically. I would continuously rewind those words in my mind at bedtime in the hope that it would suppress my fears and allow my spirit to rest before sunrise. Each day I would wake up a little stronger mentally and physically, but my immune system would get triggered quickly, and I would find my way back into the doctor's office. MS was cruel and pushed me into positions I didn't want to venture into.

I had to build a different persona to support the disease from the day I received my spinal tap. That type of pain toughened and changed my outlook on my life. My smile and laughter were now forced. Those who knew me needed to get re-introduced to me. They faced this thick blanket of a blank, bold, and hardened façade, a new and different Diana. My attitude grew stoic and rigid, like nails sliding down a chalkboard. I constantly sought out solitude. It was easier to deal with all my hurt alone, rather than being asked how I was feeling and a million times given no solution and no explanation on how to fix it. I figured out how to fake wellness enough to get by from everyone except Manmie Lea and my mother. No matter how much I was in pain, I was able to crack a sore, superficial smile. Even when I was at my worst. My facial spasms were intense—the unearthly sensation of worms crawling through, trying to break out my skin, alongside compounded migraines. I would what I thought needed to be done to stop the feeling of tingling and twitching sensation in my face. Smacking and punching myself only aggravated the spasms. They would convulse uncontrollably as if it was resisting my attempts to desensitize them; I would wash my face and then cry myself to sleep.

To help with my symptom, doctors gave me steroids. Just shy of my tenth birthday, I gained thirty pounds practically overnight. The intense steroid therapy ignited my weight gain, and MS stifled my balance which caused me to have a gait when I walked and dragged my foot. My body being introduced to steroids and a mixture of decadent, emotionally charged binge eating of processed foods only assisted in weight gain and more frequent exacerbations. No one knew the consequences of a poor diet. We thought proper medication was going to solve the problem. My lack of equilibrium made it impossible to enjoy physical activity, as did my hypersensitivity to temperature.

By age twelve, I had ballooned to a hundred and forty-five pounds. My brother had running jokes about my weight gain. He projected that I would gain ten pounds per year for every birthday. It wasn't far from the truth. Even though we all sat at the dinner table and laughed about it, it tore me apart. There were things I couldn't control, and my weight was one of them. Doctors used steroids to try to decrease inflammation and stop the number of lesions in my brain from multiplying. Such a poor balance made me anxious and uncomfortable around people, especially at my new school. I couldn't walk in a straight line, and individuals often pointed it out. I am sure my gait didn't go unnoticed, either.

I wanted to fit in and be an average child; to help me lose weight, I thought it would be a good idea to join my junior high school's dance team. I couldn't remember combinations, and I would get terrible vertigo. I thought it had to do with my weight. I took it upon myself and researched a 'good' eating *disorder*. In my pubescent mind, I wanted to learn to be bulimic or stop eating because it may prevent weight gain. I was unable to commit. My body continued through various stages of relapses and remission; I gained weight very quickly. I was taking large amounts of corticosteroids via injections. The psychological impacts of the pain and weight gain were uncanny and devastating. I overindulged with food as my pacifier to help me cope with my pain. The swelling in my brain continued, the lesions multiplied, and overwhelming stress mangled my spirit and mind. Throughout the next three years, after I was diagnosed, I would be introduced to five different medications, Interferon-Beta drugs, to help fight my relapses. Unknown to me, beta drugs lowered my immune system. I took four of them between the ages of ten and sixteen.

Few are lab-created versions of the body's illness-fighting protein. Interferon-beta drugs are called biological because they are made with living cells but formed in labs. They are all injected intramuscularly to treat adults, and a few other medicines fall into the same category. I dare not reveal names for liability's sake. Infection betas are to alleviate and stop the pain signals in the brain. The syringes were pre-filled daily auto injections half the length of my pinky.

I had no choice of which of the three parts of my body I was to jab. I began with my stomach moving to my thighs when my belly got sore. After a few dozen times, welts, hyperpigmentation, and bruises would violate my skin. That meant during gym, and I was embarrassed to wear shorts. After that, I resorted to my arms, which meant no short sleeves. My first medication was an injection, and as I staticky changed medicines, so did the needle's dosage and size. Regardless of how much encouragement I received from my parents and grandmother, I felt violated with every injection. First, It was the pain from the injection, bruising, and swelling at the injection site. The worst of it all was the side effects. I was so bewildered that I thought it was the symptoms of multiple sclerosis. I missed so many days of school because of flu-like symptoms, chronic fatigue, nausea and vomiting, headaches, soreness at the injection site, vertigo, and numbness caused by immobility. I also discovered that my chronic depression and suicidal thoughts and attempts were effects. Dosage by dosage, these meds were lowering my white blood cell count.

I faced new challenges every morning with Multiple Sclerosis that wouldn't allow me to forget how incapable and miserable I was. I was intimidated by its deceptiveness and uncertainty. Relapse after relapse, new trial drug after trial drug, I continued to sink into a deeper griev-ance. I was losing myself. My body went through immense changes in such a short time. I became introverted and recoiled while the disease began to flare and rear its ugly head. Consumed by embarrassment and hurt, I didn't want anyone to notice me and obtain knowledge that I had these visceral handicaps. Therefore, my rough exterior became the only way to keep others at a distance. My attitude became a social repel-lent. After my diagnosis, I had a new persona, and I didn't like her, but I had to keep her around so people wouldn't discover how sick I was. I just wanted to be told that one of these medications would save me.

My life hinged on my grandmother's care, prayers, constant attention, and my mother's persistence, tough love, and vigilance. Everyone else, including the doctors, filled my mind with fear and ambiguity. I carried my weary pride around like a total eclipse until I was twenty-four years old.

My heart, soul, and self-esteem felt void learning of my glim prognosis. It took two years until a neurologist gave me my diagnosis. It comforted my parents, knowing I had been diagnosed with something. What that something was, they didn't have a clear understanding, nor would I. Although Multiple Sclerosis has no cure or etiology, my parents and I were repeatedly reassured that there were treatments for the lesions and inflammation in my brain. The neurologist continued to use sizeable medical terminology and gave us no dictionary. Words like demyelination, which is the deterioration of the (myelin Seth) were unfamiliar to a pair of young black immigrant parents and a nine-year-old. The types of laboratory tests being administered, like MRI (Magnetic resonance imaging), are the imaging of the brain and or spinal cord. The list goes on. As much as I tried to retain information, it just wouldn't stick, nor was I able to maintain enough focus.

My mother constantly reminded me that I was stronger than MS. At the time, I thought *it* would do away with my entire existence. I thought I was going crazy. Regardless my mother held me to some high strict standards. She expected me to be more challenging than *it was*. I didn't have that kind of strength to fight disease; I wasn't equipped with enough knowledge.

On the other hand, my grandmother was ready to console me even if she suspected I was upset or down. I was living day by day, feeling ominous and confused. She was very profoundly empathetic. Alas, I would instead have dealt with my pain, frustration, and whatever symptoms MS would throw at me alone until I died because I knew I would be alone. I remained in the confinement of my thoughts. Solitude comforted me even though I was in my own miserable company, and my thoughts left me emotionally and mentally unavailable. At least I wouldn't have to explain why I lacked the strength to fight this unearthly battle if I fought alone. Multiple Sclerosis shrunk me mentally and emotionally.

.   My internal revolt was in full effect. I spent almost two months of ongoing diagnostic testing to being told to go home without any conclusive diagnosis. During my discharge, all I was thinking was *can I spend just a few more days?* I was not ready for this world to see me. Yet I was prepared to get out of that institution.

I spent my entire summer confined to a hospital bed – my bedroom -then my backyard. I watched for months while the outside world continued while I was being quarantined, enforced by my brother- whom my mother was dictating. I was never going to be free now. I was being held captive in my own home. It threatened every ounce of my sanity. I contemplated how to pass the time until it was time to go. I felt worthless. What life was I supposed to live if I couldn't enjoy the simple things?

MS was nonexistent in our family. I am the only one in my known lineage to have a such ailment., Even with newer technology, it is less than 1 percent of children with MS, including black children. The are many other childhood autoimmune disorders with similar symptoms and characteristics- such as Lyme disease, migraine, stroke, Lupus, and Vitamin B-12 Deficiency, to name a few that were in the running. These diagnoses were on the table for two years before I was given Multiple Sclerosis as a firm and final diagnosis.

My frustrations started to amplify. P.O.M.S wasn't even a medical term back then. I began to familiarize myself with medical terminology superficially. My name became synonymous with medical terms. The doctor's delivery of what was happening to my body and how to treat it was weak and left me numb. MS introduced me to realities I wasn't ready to encounter nor couldn't accept because of the fragility of being so young. Pediatricians aren't familiar with MS because they are not expecting to see it in children, let alone black children. I understand why my pediatrician hastily told my mother to take me to the emergency room. However, because of increased awareness of childhood MS since I was finally diagnosed in early 2001, after visiting three different doctors –Charcot, if he were alive, would have raved about the advancements in modern neurology and technology- but for me, these achievements just weren't enough. The fact that I was such an anomaly never sat right with me. My narratives were never told, highlighted, or seen. The number of children diagnosed with MS is rapidly growing, and better treatments are being sought on a case-by-case basis, but none are good enough to cure it. Instead, they leave children co-dependent on treatment or open another can of worms that causes more symptoms that aren't necessarily affiliated with MS.

Although most days felt worse than others, my heart continued to darken. I thought my demise would be around the corner. I was unaware that my worst days hadn't even dawned on me yet.

Weeks after my release, I was still perplexed and out of sorts about my new reality. I was a victim of my circumstances with no foundation to stand on. My self-doubt echoed like my migraines. My anger grew more significant than my stature. I quickly became subservient to the unknown. The fear of the unknown combined with the muscle aches, facial spasms, numbness, anxiety, tremors, and judgment left me irrational, easily irritated, and depressed. Filled with fear and remorse, I harbored a lot of angst and anger. I did have the comprehension of where not to place my energy.

Regardless of how sick I felt, my mother urged me mentally and physically to get out of bed. My grandmother nurtured me spiritually and emotionally; to say the least, I was divided. My mother parented with an iron fist, and when *she* wasn't available, my brother was my honorary disciplinarian and warden. I misunderstood their tough love as not being fond of me because I was the *sick one* – immediately, I thought my family had a vendetta against me, and there went my imagination again!

I know my parents always made my medical decisions in my best interest. I couldn't acknowledge their sacrifices at the time. My mind was warped in such turmoil. I was in between furious and depressed and blinded by self-pity. That left me unequipped and irrational; most judgments were made without understanding why. I was too delicate and weak, but neither my mother nor grandmother would give up on me, nor would they allow me to give up on myself. My spirit was vulnerable. It was hard to acknowledge that my mother would spare no expense to keep me healthy.

These were unsolvable riddles left for me to figure out on my own. My decision-making was fueled by anxiety and fear of what would become if I didn't surrender.

Destiny was an unfavorable concept to me. My end seemed dark, near, cold, and empty. No one would be able to understand the infractions that I was up against. I would have horrific dreams of the children mocking my face. The students wouldn't be able to stomach my appearance, for even I found my reflection repulsive and hideous. Experiencing Hemi's facial spasm was a skeevy feeling. When I looked in the mirror, I saw my nerves jumping out of my skin like tiny worms trying to escape my flesh. Though it passed in less than a year, it was a slow and grueling feeling that even the doctors couldn't unearth or make disappear. I was apprehensive as well about the medication, but like every great addict, I awaited my next fix, hoping it would help my problems go away. Without it, I could not make it through the hallways of my private Catholic junior high school. Everyone at my school came from affluent, white catholic backgrounds. Less than eight percent were multicultural students; black, Spanish, and south pacific islanders.

My differences shrank me. The children fed into that energy, and I quickly became ostracized. I was failing tests and watching other children advance. Who would be friends to befriend someone in my current state? The chronic episodes were documented one after the other and came at me like clockwork.

Though my symptoms remitted, and I relapsed several times for all to witness within two years, despite the diagnosis, I remained resilient. When my body went into remission, it was short-lived. I thought I was on my way to being cured; my exterior continued to fade; my hair began to fall out with every injection. My flare-ups (exacerbations) would sometimes last months. The tingling, pinching, twitching, and Hemi facial muscle spasms dragged on for months. I wanted to hide the symptoms of Bell's Palsy from the world, which made me feel utterly repulsive and tortured me mentally. That was one of my worse symptoms besides my gait because they were both physically seen. It took a toll on my confidence and consciousness. I didn't want to be around my family, let alone other children my age, or in the eye of the public. The spark that I once held in my soul began to slip away. Rigid and tired, I would get dressed up in my uniform and go to school in the rain, sleet, and snow regardless of how monstrous I felt or thought my reflection was. I mustered what little courage I had. I was a broken little brown girl with an ominous crooked smile.

7

❖

Lessons on Pediatric MS

"Stress is caused only if you commit to the problems weighing you down."
~Diana Lea M

I started junior high school fall of '99, weeks after being discharged from the hospital. The transition happened so quickly that I couldn't grasp nor address what precisely what I was being thrown into. My mind was out of sorts. If I wasn't falling asleep during class, going home early from school because of chronic pain and numbness, or violently vomiting my lunch because of vertigo. I was losing my mind over the sheer embarrassment of stumbling in my penny loafers or someone bearing witness to my disfigured face.

September 11, 2001, was the day I wished I had played the absent card, but my resiliency took center stage that morning. Manmie Lea helped me get ready most mornings; this day was no different. Although my mother was my wake-up call at 4 am before she left out for work, Mama Lea woke up before the sun in prayer, meditation, and coffee. I would float back to sleep and hope to wake up on time. By 4:30 am, my grandmother would walk up the stairs and start my count down for the school bus that I had to walk two blocks to catch. Some days I was reluctant. My father or a neighbor would drive me to the bus stop. I would drag my spirit out of bed then my body would follow. Mama Lea fueled my heart with her charisma, "Put your big girl pants on," she exclaimed in creole, encouraging me to get ready a bit quicker. She would press my uniform early morning, which she washed by hand the night before.

My movement was slow, repetitive, and sloth-like. I arrived at the school bus by the skin of my teeth. The weather was hot and humid for a mid-September morning in Long Island, New York. I caught the bus and arrived at school within an hour with a splitting headache and exhaustion. The entire student and facility body sat through morning prayer and announcements. As the first period began, all was seemingly fine until 8:46 am, when America's history changed forever. That morning, an airplane was hijacked and flown into one of the World Trade Center Towers. Literally minutes away from where my father had worked, and just moments after, another airplane hit the other tower. Minor details of the hijacking began to unravel. The teachers rolled out the classroom television and projected America's chaos. Right there, we witnessed a ripple in history on the television screen. My heart was filled with sadness. I felt this before, but it was different when other people felt similar sentiments. As my country was in complete disarray, and so was I. I was stressed over my father's whereabouts. My worries overshadowed my pain. My eyes were swelling up with tears, thinking about what may have happened to him.

The usually quiet hallways of my high school were filled with the cries and clamor of the administration and the student body. The intensity built as the moments of uncertainty and calamity resonated throughout the building. The teacher began to pull students one by one out of class until my high school decided on an early emergency dismissal. Sometimes, I would lounge or sit in the office for hours until the day's end or my flare subsided. Today felt like the world was flaring up.

My uneasiness continued to fester throughout the morning. To top it off, one of the students pointed out the elephant in the classroom and shouted, *"Diana, my eyelids have been twitching all morning. Does that mean I have what you got?"* I gave her a great eye roll and sighed as I looked down. My pulse began to race, and to try not to make eye contact with her as my blood curdled; I gave her a cold stare. I shook my head and murmured, *"no."* All that heavy, negative energy hovered over me, which triggered tightness in my chest. It was hard to breathe, but I didn't complain or alert anyone. I wanted to say much more to her, but I was at a loss for words. I thought they could see my problem, but no *one cared*. It lasted the entire way home. I was embarrassed more than upset. I sat in the back of the school bus, hoping I would disappear. It wasn't a smooth or silent bus ride home. I couldn't fall asleep on the bus and didn't own a cell phone; therefore, I could not check up on my father's whereabouts.

The whole bus ride, I was engulfed by a bubble of anxiety thinking about my father. My distress made me feel heavy, weary, and tired. When I arrived home, terrorists had hijacked another aircraft and flown into the Pentagon building in Washington, D.C. The nation was in a state of emergency and complete turmoil.

My worry and exhaustion rested on my face. Emotionally, mentally, and physically, I was ready to snap. I braced myself as I hobbled home, walked in, and found my grandmother cooking a storm in the kitchen. She didn't speak much English nor watch much television, so it was clear she was oblivious to the news. As I stepped into the kitchen, she stopped cooking; I took a big inhale as she reached over for her glasses, looked boldly into my eyes, and scanned my face. She smiled, and then I exhaled, and she went back to stirring the pot. Usually, her energy would wipe away all my pain and the day's transgressions. I looked forward to some calm and home-cooked food. Mama tried to be particular about what she fed me: not too starchy or greasy, and a lot of salads, greens, and proteins. She could cater to me regardless of what was made for anyone else. My Caribbean ancestry allowed spices to immerse in the air.

I dropped my backpack on the dining room table. I doubled back into the kitchen, and I slowly approached her. She paused and kissed me gingerly on my forehead. I hugged her as tightly as I could, and my chest compressed. I asked her in Creole, *"where was papa?"* She shrugged and told me he should be home by seven. I shrugged and said to her that I was going upstairs to my room to change out of my uniform and call my mother, that would be back. I walked sluggishly toward the stairs, and I was finally able to make finally made my way up without taking a break. I lugged myself to my bedroom and locked the door behind me. I would never return from my room if I didn't promise Mammie Lea that I would come back to eat supper. I would rather sleep on an empty stomach.

Ready to lock myself in the darkness, I turned on my air conditioner and turned off my bedroom lights. My eyes were beginning to become more sensitive with every passing day. I collapsed on my bed, feeling like I had just run a 10k marathon. Exhaustion, sadness, and frustrations filled my spirit to my core. As I lay on the bed, I scrambled to take my uniform off. It bothered me severely that I didn't have the stamina to do minor things. I gave up, as my fatigue was malicious. It was senseless trying to come to terms with something I did not understand. MS is a vicious disease, and I couldn't comprehend to what capacity its savagery would do to my body, let alone the correct way to pronounce it. Frustrated and sweating profusely, I began to sob when I felt my legs cramping and seizing up underneath me. Pins and needles were marching up and down the right side of my lower limbs and bottom. I just wanted to seek refuge from the pain. The sensation ran from my tippy toes up to the right side of my face. I curled into a ball and continued to break into a wall of tears, turning my headache into an ice-cold migraine.

My leg spasms became unbearable as I lay quietly, panicking, scared, and vulnerable in a sea of mental despair. As I was sobbing, the muscles in my eye and lips twitched and flickered like a dying light bulb. I didn't utter a sound. I remained pained in silence so I wouldn't draw attention to myself. I didn't want to worry Mammie Lea.

I managed to sit up and stretched out my legs as I n tried to wiggle my toes, but they wouldn't move. Thoughts of my father not making it home for dinner raced through my mind. I leaned over and then physically pinched my toes. They were numb to the touch. I began hitting my legs violently as my legs because they were completely relaxed. I threw my torso back down in my bed, cradled my pillow to my face, and screamed into it as I began kicking my legs. Minutes passed as I lay and closely followed the digital clock on my dresser across from my bed with my weary eyes. My sight was the only sense that seemed to work. My face began convulsing. Cramps and spasms began to numb my forehead to my mouth suddenly. I could barely unzip my romper and tried to take it off unsuccessfully. Wiping away my tears with the edge of the bottom of my romper, my frustration grew, yet I wouldn't give up.

I ended up pulling it up over my head. There was no want to settle. I was committed to regaining my senses to get back down those stairs and being with my grandmother again. Maybe she could call my mom to find out where my father was. Manmie Lea and my father weren't on the best-speaking terms back then since he asked her to leave a year before I got sick.

Thoughts raced through my mind trying to figure out how my day had become so daunting. I wondered where I had gone wrong. I was decent this morning. My body was becoming uncontrollable, as well as my emotions. I was overwhelmed by all these feelings. I didn't understand how to cope or what to fix these attacks.

I began concentrating all my energy and strength to get out of bed. I turned into the darkness, *myself*. Regardless of the lights already being off, as time progressed, my room seemed to become even darker and more daunting as the daylight faded. Yet, I never knew this type of darkness could even exist. I could just lay in the still of the night as tears fell, and I cried my way to sleep.

I woke up to the same piercing migraine and nausea as my

grandmother was yodeling my name up the stairway for supper. I tried to sleep off the migraine I had brought home from school. Flustered and angry, I was still determined and felt this attempt would be different. I called back my grandmother. I was starving, so much so that the nausea was overwhelming.

I knew what my body wouldn't allow me to do, but my mind was rather persistent and motivated. My heart yearned to get back down to my grandmother. I was sure she had tea brewing and waiting for me. Her herbal teas had a way of making me feel almost revitalized and soothing my spirit. I needed this stale and incompetent feeling to melt away. There wasn't an ounce of positivity that flowed through my body at this point, just dark thoughts and the sheer determination to get back to her. Since my release from the hospital, I began to neglect and deprive myself of essential nourishment and necessities. Happiness didn't matter more. I was a broken brown girl suffering in silence. It was only when my grandmother was near or when she called my name that I found a little peace, joy, and warmth in her voice. Her prayers and consciousness held my hope. Yet I still couldn't find the strength to rise and get to her.

My struggle to get back down for supper had me thinking less about my father and more focused on getting back down to Mammie Lea. I became relaxed, and all the tension in my body dissipated. I closed my eyes. I thought long and hard about what waited for me on the dining room table and began to repeat one of my grandmother's favorite prayers to myself. I decided to move and thought I had to exaggerate my movements and be more calculated in how I tried getting out of bed.

I meditated, committed to the execution of the movement of my legs. I didn't care about the fuzzy feeling in my face any longer or the pin and needles. Seconds then minutes passed, and the tingling sensation in my face, legs, and arms got more robust. The stress surged throughout my body. Trying to be an ordinary girl seemed so costly and made me want to give up. My ongoing trials resulted in consistent errors, which exhausted me. I knew I had to relax. My mother arrived home; I heard my grandmother and her talking downstairs.

Moments later, my grandmother yodeled again from the bottom of the wooden staircase. I thought she was about to make her way to my room. This triggered further anxiety. Then, I remembered I had forgotten to call my mom. I didn't want her to know I was like this. I knew she would like to take me to the doctor immediately. I didn't want to work her up, and I didn't want to return to the hospital. I yelled back and told my grandmother that I was coming and resting a bit more.

After a while, I became tranquil and fully relaxed, my muscles allowing the tension to flow through and release from my body again. I was relentless. I reopened my eyes, slid off my stockings, and massaged my legs. One by one lifted my legs to my chest, hugged my leg, and then my leg to the forehead. I was flexible, although I could no longer dance. The pins and needles sensation funneled down my legs to my toes. I wiggled my toes and was able to feel them. With much persistence, I began to stabilize. I tried to grip the cold ground beneath me with my bare feet. The lack of sensation caused me to fall short. I couldn't feel the ground. Then like a sloth, I slithered slowly off my bed and lowered myself to the floor. With both knees planted on the ground and me holding on to the side of my bed, I tried to get up and walk.

Although I didn't have enough sensation to walk, I tried to glide across my glossy wooden floors by overthinking my every step and dragging the heavier foot to place one foot in front of the other. Still, my stride again seemed forced and stiff, like ice skates gliding on the pavement. *Forward*, I thought, moving nowhere until I landed face-first. My mother then called my name. I inhaled deeply. *Hi mommy*, I yelled, hoping she heard me.

My foot continued to drag. The drag of the foot is clinically known as foot drop, which is a high gait when walking, and I made a loud enough thud to make my grandmother yell if I was okay. I assured her I was and that I was coming, but honestly, I was exhausted.

My spirit was broken, and I felt almost defeated. My nerves rattled and echoed me. Chills ran through my body cold, yet I was sweating. I found myself stuck between great walls of frustration. My anger grew even more intensely as my belly raged because I was hungry. My emotions were mangled, bruised, battered, and anger began to boil over. All I wanted was my family together and a good meal after such a catastrophic day.

I rose to my knees and began to slip back down as my nerves continued to rattle, but I finally caught hold of my weight and could lean against the table for support. I continued to push my way through my pain and exhaustion. I reached forward, grabbed the doorknob, and turned it to the right. I pulled the door open with a crackling voice and yelped, "Did papa call yet?" Manmie Lea said he called and would be home soon. There was terrible traffic getting out of the city.

Rattled by anxiety, my voice quivered, trying to grip my nerves to answer my grandmother. I gathered myself and went down for dinner. After everyone arrived home safely that night, I lay exhausted, but my mind did not let me rest the night. I stayed up, analyzing all the alternatives that could have happened. This was just another one of my sleepless nights.

8

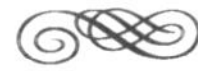

F.O.M.O -Fear of
Missing Out

"If you want to keep a secret, you must hide it from yourself."
George Orwell

My teacher's gut instinct changed the trajectory of the rest of my life. She saw something no one, not even my parents, grandmother, or next-door neighbor, who usually cleaned my face before carpooling with some other children from the neighborhood. Auntie Dawn, as I respectfully called her, was of no relation to me but looked after me. She was like a great-aunt. Full of wisdom and got along with my grandmother; though they didn't speak the same language, they managed to communicate well. She fed and nurtured me as if we were related. When I was in elementary school, she allied with my grandmother and mother to ensure I went to school every morning. Then on Sundays, I would look forward to Sunday school with Dawn or church with grandma. Either one was an experience where I could worship in song and dance, learn, and enjoy with other children my age. MS stole those fond moments from me and left me estranged from my faith, as if my life had no meaning.

If it wasn't for my six-grade teacher, I don't think my story would be half as interesting. After diagnosis, my reality didn't set in. The pain was draining mentally and emotionally as I was already physically distraught. I struggled with my faith and slowly turned my back on God. What I was learning in school differed from what I was brought up learning from my grandmother, and Sunday school with auntie Dawn taught me. It felt like an eternal nightmare of confusion. I didn't understand how my place in the world was stolen from me and was turning me out to be a misfit. "If Jesus loved me, this I know. Was it because the bible told me so? Or did my school bind me to faith in something foreign to me? What with all a lie? I couldn't understand why this disease was so ambiguous. It wrecked my mind. I lived in a constant state of torment, trying to construct how did this possibly happen to me. What did I do to bear such an anomaly? Multiple Sclerosis ruined the ideals I set for myself and built new expectations of me. My whimsical dreams evaporated into thin air as entitlement overshadowed my reality and left me with a vastness of emptiness. I never knew entitlement was such a dirty word. It conflicted with what my mother taught me about doctors' orders, in the sense that how sick was I to sit back and allow things to unfold? It seemed as if doctors didn't care for the quality of my life. I was to continue with the routine without too many questions. I tried to find another way, but there weren't many options available. I knew I had to take on new adversities, yet I was still fearful and didn't know how or what to do. I was barely a teenager, unable to take on such responsibility and quickly.

I was stuck in the summer of 1999, which crippled me and left me walking through a dark, desolate, twisted, and vulnerable path. My then juvenile immune system and mind were not prepared to fight. My body already had a mix of cocktails, which had many adverse effects. How am I supposed to combat something of such a great multitude unarmed?

I thought I was losing my mind as I tried to get a handle on balancing my emotions and teenage hormones. From missed menstrual cycles to heavy bleeding for over eight days and crying spells at the drop of a dime, I couldn't get a grip on my weird emotional and physical roller-coaster. I was in denial for so long, and in the back of my mind, I knew my feelings had to be justified or I was going insane. My emotions came to me in tsunami-like waves. The day I walked through those hospital emergency room doors, my heart crumbled, and I was hit by the first wave and left on the floor shattered in pieces. The doctors tried to piece me back together in time for my first day of school, but I'd never be the same again. My parents, brother, and doctors kept me under close observation for the rest of my adolescence and teenage years. MS extracted my joy. I no longer became interested in the things I grew up loving because my energy was focused on the pain. I would never get to live and enjoy the transition from elementary school to junior high, childhood to pre-teen. It was as if the space in time was a complete blur. Everything moved faster than my mind could comprehend

I knew I had no choice for the first time as MS stripped me of my liberty. My oasis of hope and joy ran dry. I was fruitless. My hurt was adorned on my sleeve, and as I got older, my subconscious became so vulnerable and sensitive that people could easily pick at my fragile ego. MS weakened my body, mind, faith, and spirit. I became haunted by the fact that I would never be able to share in my peers' memories at graduation. This feeling echoed throughout my adolescence and my adulthood. I buried my angst deep inside and allowed them to suffocate me.

Diagnosis with MS has been the most uncomfortable life-long adjustment and seemed impossible for me. Being misdiagnosed for almost two years led to many uncertainties and a loss of hope. We were ready to accept nearly any diagnosis. Early detection also led to early intervention, which gave me, in hindsight, a better prognosis; unfortunately, I didn't see it that way. My pain blinded me.

I'm not a parent yet, but I can never imagine what my mother, father, and grandmother endured with me being sick. My siblings also had to deal with many versions of me because I didn't know how to deal with MS. I thought my diagnosis would put our minds at ease, but it didn't. Not in the least. It made me want to place blame and put me severely on edge. It was easy to personify negativity in every part of my life because I lived it. I focused it on the people I was closest to, mainly my grandmother and mom. My mother never treated me like I was handicapped or sick, although she always kept me under a microscope.

I thought she wanted to suffocate the last bit of freedom I felt had left. Depression began to dictate my life. I saw every standard my mother held me to be another way for her to control my life, even when she wasn't present because my older brother became my foreman. Sacha kept me under constant surveillance, ready to submit daily reports to her. Multiple Sclerosis took over my life, and no one could help me but myself.

9

A child with a Dove

"I couldn't run from the pain, so I ran towards it" ~ Sean Carter, *aka Jay-Z.*

It began as a bottomless downward spiral with no ending in sight. I'd come face to face with a dance that I couldn't master. The perplexity of my symptoms postponed my willingness to accept my diagnosis. Though giving up wasn't an option, we anticipated a diagnosis for two years, and to be told there was no cure was heartbreaking. Medications were placed in front of my parents and me disguised as if they were presents on Christmas morning. The treatment options granted me were worse than the truth that I have an incurable disease. I honestly think I wouldn't be better off if I hadn't taken medication. Then I sometimes wonder, if I didn't, would it even matter? Would I have saved some of the most traumatic moments of my life? My feeling of relief rests in the fact that I am informed. I'm no less opposed to medication than I opposed to its side effects. They have never added to my joy or the quality of my life. If my mother weren't stern with me, I wouldn't have the will to stand up for myself and stop treatment.

I can't blame all my emotional instabilities and inadequacies, but I don't listen to the sciences; I hear and digest them. MS made me grow intensely analytical, and that is in all aspects of life. I observe, and I deduce rather than observe and induce. It lessened my ability to get hurt and feel lesser pain. I was rushing to experience life because my concept of living was cut short. Not one of my decisions didn't have a consequence. I singled handed, became an assessor to MS, and began sabotaging my life. Lessons of value, morals, and beliefs that I still carry with me today. Yes, I mostly stayed home because of MS, but once I was out, what I craved was mine for the moment; I wanted to experience not worrying about the consequence. Multiple sclerosis became my scapegoat.

I skipped school to avoid being bullied and ostracized. I was going to foreign cities outside my Long Island limits. Sometimes alone, others with almost equally vigilante classmates. My grades continued to worsen on the border of failure. As if I wasn't already being punished, my brother found an excellent way to punish me. I thought my life was *punishment enough. How can you punish me any more than God was doing? It was most certainly the worse of the two evils because I couldn't keep up, regardless of whether* I was present or not in school. Even when I received a week of in-school suspension when another student accosted me, I wasn't fazed, I couldn't stand up for myself, but I hit her with a textbook in self-defense. To my surprise, my mother advocated for me, hoping for less severe punishment. That altercation was followed by detention for a few Saturdays and demerits (a mark or stakes awarded to a person for fault or offense); besides the lump on my forehead, I didn't care much. Lying to your parents is never a good decision, and I felt that my mother supported me in several instances when I didn't deserve it.

Anger changes people in massive proportion. Anger clogs and impairs judgment. It impoverished my soul and bought me out of character. I was doing things that embarrassed my parents and most certainly embarrassed me. With no care, I continued to rationalize my incompetent and irrational behavior. My diagnosis was like three dots on a fresh toe tag. My clock was ticking, and I felt like I could die anytime. I figured that I needed to start living. I was impractical with how I dealt with MS for over a decade, but I knew no better. I couldn't get a handle on how to reangle any facet of it. I began to exploit the unexplainable instead of starving it or looking for answers.

I had to pack up my dance shoes and bury them with much regret and sadness. My legs were useless to me without balance and coordination, and so was my mind. My dance lessons replaced doctor visits, syringes, chronic pains, and endless medical exams. I struggled quietly internally when I was in public throughout my life. I felt inferior and insecure. I tried to cover those feelings up by being rude, bold, and loud at home. Taking out my anxiety, anger, frustration, and confusion on my family, especially on my mother, grandmother, and sometimes even my baby sister. When my behavior got out of hand, and I became intolerable, my mother made my brother instill the fear of God in me. My mother was stricken with hypertension in her early thirties. She didn't want to stress. Therefore, she let my brother do the "dirty" work and set forth punishments instead of precedence., *I don't care. I'm going to die anyway. What else can you take away from me that I haven't already lost? Disgruntled, nothing could have been worse than the hell I felt I already was living in.*

I had outgrown my backyard and wanted to experience what was beyond my gate of solitary confinement, but my brother wouldn't let me out of his sight. I became resentful. When the weather was the nicest, my antics kept me indoors. It added sheer insult to all the many disadvantages plaguing me. I thought I was entitled to get my way regardless of my behavior. *After all, I'm going to die; I should be able to be as irrational as I want to be.* Not even my grandmother could fill the void that was inside me. I felt helpless and torn. I would alleviate my pain with food—binge eating, even when my grandmother prepared me my unique healthier meal options. Unsatisfied, I'd figure out a way to go up the block and buy cheesy fries, spicy chicken sandwiches with cheese, nuggets, and a frosty or tell my dad to bring me home pizza.

I struggled for over a decade with these horrible habits, yet I would torture myself for years. It became the drug of my choice. Inner turmoil and handicaps allowed food to continue to fill that void. MS didn't allow for minor adjustments. Instead, it thrashed me into a world filled with inevitable challenges. Finding a balance between my scholastics, this disease, and any social life was impossible. My physicians told me I might never graduate, which would be expected if I didn't. That's when the life I imagined for myself seemed utterly unattainable. My mother always told me to stay strong and not to get overly excited. She imagined it would cause me to flare up or exacerbate. How can I not get frustrated and upset, and all I heard was the word of my inabilities? I insisted on doing and going against my mother's wishes. Intentionally, I began to overcompensate for things I thought I would lose the chance to experience. Over time, it significantly impacted my overall mental, emotional, and physical health. My goals were extinguished. Birthdays were my worst days, filled with emptiness and lonely thoughts. There was nothing to celebrate; nowhere I could go. I would wonder why I am still alive. Where did the joy go? My mother wouldn't allow me to attend or join any events at school. My limitations went beyond what MS handed me. I felt constantly displaced, making it easier to become a victim and ostracized. Quickly, I became the prime target of bullying and harassment from other children. Picked on and tactically torn apart and left in tears daily by other children about my weight and inabilities, I didn't experience happiness in school or at home. I kept crying for help, but no one could hear me.

My high school was very ornate. The entryway was grand and lavish, adorned with giant statues. I quickly became unimpressed by its grandeur. High above the tall glass doors leading into the interior of the building were carved the words "One Heart and One mind" and "W.W.J.D (What would Jesus do). Only if they knew Jesus was a black man would that make them indifferent. The entry hall walls were lined with old white dead men called brother and father. It was eerie and ominous, especially when classes were in session, and I walked down the hallway alone with my head studying the ground so I won't fall. Focusing on my penny loafers as I walked awkwardly on the waxed marbled floors that led past the foyer and the glass solarium/ greenhouse. As I made my way to the nurse's office down the hall, I passed its inhabitants, peacocks, other delicate exotic birds, and sizeable coy fish. Stained glass windows and cathedral ceilings became part of my nightmares. The grades were divided into three floors. The lower floor housed the middle school grades six through eight. The top two floors housed the upper-class student. Grades nine and ten were on the second floor. The eleventh and twelfth graders occupied the top floor.

The entire school would participate in the morning prayer service on the rollout television screen or projector. My high school had its television station. It was mandatory to say the Lord's prayer at the beginning of every period. I would try to pep talk myself before starting my school day because there wasn't a prayer in the world that would stop me from falling asleep. Most days out of the school year, I would get called for early dismissal or sit in the nurse's office. My frequent exacerbations caused me to go to regular neurologist appointments more than I attended class.

The teacher's and students' curiosity began to peak. I was too embarrassed to explain my secret or how I felt to the doctors and administration, let alone my peers. My absences from school debunked the truth about having excused absences; regardless of how bad my flare-up or exacerbation was, I had to keep my grades up. The teachers held me accountable for any missed assignments. My parents did their part; I felt it was my duty to do mine. They were consistent with always paying my tuition on time. I couldn't let my grades suffer for fear of getting summer school. I often felt obligated to explain myself because of peer pressure. I was caught between doing what was best for me and becoming a people pleaser, trying to find where I could fit in.

I thought I had justification for doing poorly in my classes, which was reflected in my behavior and scholastics. I would do enough damage to get reprimanded but not ever enough to get expelled. I nervously waited for my report card every three months, shaking in panic. Having trimesters instead of semesters was constant pressure on my mind. It gave me less time to redeem myself in between marking periods. My mother only required that I attend school and get good grades while following doctors' protocols. She warned me that summer school wasn't optional, nor was it a failure.

Summer school cost three hundred dollars per class per week on top of the nearly eight-thousand-dollar tuition my parents were already paying. I never understood the point of sending me to private school when I was always absent. Our public schools were fine institutions. My older siblings attended the neighboring schools, which were only blocks away from our home. Regarding school matters, MS seemed less of a factor for everyone, including myself. It was never enough for me not to pass my classes, and I had to keep up by any means necessary. I was miserable, Multiple Sclerosis made me feel as if my mom was asking for the world, and I desperately wanted to do better in school and focus, but I simply couldn't. I was barely passing any of my classes. My fear of failure and anxiety were projected in all that I did. I walked around with a chip on my shoulder. I was doing so poorly that no test quiz nor assignment could redeem my inadequacies. I thought I could be as astute as the other students. I sat in front of the class, slept earlier, and got proper rest, but nothing worked.

I went from elaborate and ambitious dreams of attending the prestigious Juilliard School of Arts and wanting to dance at the Apollo to trying to survive and get through one more day. I loved tap dancing, which was my favorite art form. I emulated legends like Debbie Allen and Gregory Oliver Hines, noted African American dancers, singers, and actors. I would look forward to one day being a part of New York's world-renowned Radio Music Christmas Spectacular. Once I was diagnosed, all those doors slammed shut in my face. Weary, I felt defeated, and the feeling only persisted. I struggled with the desperation of wanting to be seen and hiding my MS. Ashamed and chronically pained, the confusion funneled this overcast of loss in the world. I became so wrapped up in what I couldn't do that I had no interest in what I was able to accomplish. The drugs kept me feeling helpless because of the ongoing side effects. Desperately, I wanted alleviation as I felt as if I was suffocating.

There is no coincidence that many of my memories after diagnosis are unclear. The intensity of the traumas I experienced compounded into mire fractions of a larger-than-life battle. Detached, I struggled to find my way. My intentions became smeared and scattered. Although it's hard to recount the amount of pressure and angst I felt trying to hide my sickness from the public, it was almost impossible. As much as I wanted to be invisible, I also craved and needed to be seen and understood. I was among the few black children at a prestigious private Catholic high school. The minority population was minuscule; I was even more under a microscope than I understood. My school was the end-all of high-priced privileged education on Long Island, New York. It was an honor for my mother that I was accepted, and at the same instance, it was my hell.

Socially awkward and anxious, I still tried to be present as the lack thereof my cognitive abilities would not allow me to. I was reluctant to engage with most of my schoolmates in any positive manner. I told tall tales to stay current and relevant but ended up in needless gossip. I felt like an outcast because I was trying to evade my illness to keep up with my peers, craving inclusion. I tried out for a dance but couldn't keep up with the prerequisites, so I had to bow out. I was naive and foolish. I lost my perspective and couldn't find my point of view.

Amidst the shuffle, one thing was constant; my love of dance and music because my mother, grandmother, and father always played music in our home Saturdays and Sundays. They loved to dance, which helped me through much of my journey. Music was a constant conduit of expression. Music helped me cope as I continued through my journey. After my first hospitalization, before I began middle school, the neurologists placed certain restrictions on my abilities, which played a large part in my insecurities, displacement, and entitlement. I couldn't retain many of my motor, coordination, balance, and muscle memory.

MS placed an abrupt end to my dance career. I fathomed; at least I could listen to music and dream. Music took my mind off and allowed me to reflect on positive times. Yet, the fact that I could no longer dance broke me. My life lost much meaning when I could no longer move as I loved to. Listening to music granted me hoped when everything seemed lost. With that, I held on to one day at a time. Maybe I would be able to dance again. That is, if MS didn't kill me first.

Now and then, a glimmer of hope would occur, and as fast as it came, MS would remind me that it was bigger than me. I could have sworn the medicines worked until my nerves began to convulse in my face, arms, and legs. My fits were the worse. My legs would give up right underneath me in mid-walk or movement without notice. These episodes would happen in waves for years, anytime, and place.

In the beginning, it was just the music, crafted beautiful poetry carried with the accent of the downbeat and a neat high hat. Early introduction to music as a baby allowed me to continue to keep my creative juices flowing. As I grew older, my taste in music eventually diversified. My palette personally matured and developed. I went from liking whatever my elders liked to bridging the gap between listing to Kompa and my generational music. My musical taste was crafted in the place that raised me, good old New York and Haiti.

I view my shortcomings as life's lessons. Changing that mindset took me from being a social introvert to being able to come to terms with Multiple Sclerosis and its dynamic diabolical symptoms, which made me feel like a leper. Researching and experimenting allowed me to become more confident in my discovery. It was like a light bulb went off in my head. This disease has been referred to as a snowflake in many articles, books, and doctors' offices. It affirmed everything I had been thinking for almost a decade. Sean Carter (aka. Jay Z's) lyrics seemed relevant to what had been happening for most of my life. "Hard Knock Life" was another album he masterminded with the sampling of *"Annie,"* my favorite musical. I picked apart the lyrics, "instead *of treated, we get tricked," which* resonated with me.

It was the invasion of the body snatchers, and I was hosting. Every time I walked into the doctor's office, I didn't get treated; instead, another medication was brought up as if it was the resolution to my problem, which was far from the truth. Whenever I felt okay, I partially had a handle on my situation. MS always reminded me and kicked me when I was coasting on my silver lining. I was told to keep out of extreme temperatures, which was hard to do in New York. I would search for freedom, but I got reprehended by my mother and then punished by my brother. She would be distraught at me when I would want to resist taking new medications. Not to mention, she would be disappointed when I skipped school.

She didn't understand how I was feeling and that fact. Doctors acted like the drugs they were administering were the only things that could save my life; therefore, we believed them. They fed me drugs and let me figure out everything else alone, with no GPS to help me navigate. It was rare that I would think about leaving my home. I began making irrational decisions by skipping school. One second, I had the energy to go to school, but then I would find my way to Coney Island by bus and train, but then not remember how to get back. Looking back, I was living so dangerously, and no one knew how disturbed I was. Mentally, I couldn't adjust to either the social changes or the physical challenges I was up against. My circumstances were overwhelming, and they began to consume me. Being sick was a burden because I couldn't connect with many of my peers. Mentally and physically, I was exhausted, and my symptoms came and gone as my heart grew weary and weak, and I continued to shrink spiritually. Time seemed to have stopped for me, and I didn't know how to cope. I was stuck in limbo.

Unable to escape the multitude of physical restrictions and emotional rollercoasters that kept tormenting me night and day. The burden of the neurologist's lists of do's and don'ts lamented on my mind. In time, the list lengthened. I became unstable, cold, withdrawn, and utterly exhausted at eleven. Physically, the pressure of waking up daily was a task. I couldn't relieve myself of the strengths that disabled my physical shell, mental, and emotional. I grew to let my handicaps consume my identity. My adolescence became a fight to get back to just being Diana again. The doctors wanted me to accept that I was a broken black little girl. They failed to realize that the women I came from were black and whole.

Though I felt severely inflicted by MS and its complications, that just wasn't who I was.

It took away my time and aged me quickly without remorse, and it seemed like doctors expected me to be ok with that idea. As my body became maimed and lame, my heart also wilted away. I started believing that I must have done something wrong to affect how my life was tainted, disrupted, and obstructed. As the years went by, I concluded that death was inevitable.

10

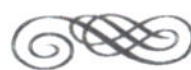

Weeping Girl

Chapter 10 **Weeping Girl**
"I wasn't made for reality, but life came and found me"- Fernando Pessoa.

Hours into my first hospital stay, I began to develop numbness and tingling sensation in my face. In the following weeks, the tingling and numbness turned into partial paralysis of my right side, which traveled throughout my face, fingers, legs, and toes. My body felt as if it was on the wrong channel, and the antenna was only giving off snowy-like static. I began suffering from sensory deficiency, extreme fatigue, weakness, and vertigo. As time continued, so did newer symptoms like twitching and spasticity in my legs and arms. My disease became highly aggressive, and so were my treatment options. We were praying that the steroids would cure me. I learned that it was because the doctors didn't have a precise diagnosis. Therefore, they gave me a generic drug to alleviate my symptoms. There weren't sufficient cases to compare me to. I learned that I was seen as an anomaly decades after my diagnosis.

Doctors couldn't correctly treat a rarity like mine because my narrative hadn't been included in any study.

I didn't understand what was going on internally. The age of reason hadn't dawned upon me yet; there, I couldn't justify my misery except that I must have been disobedient. Locked in my sterile jail cell, I hadn't any option but to comply with doctors' orders. I grew angry and sad as my summer ended abruptly. It would be a week before I began middle school in unchartered territory when I was discharged from the hospital. When I arrived home, I didn't just feel like a stranger; I felt like a stranger in my own body.

My siblings would constantly stop and stare at me. My parents were also in my face frequently as if they carried answers. I already knew I was disfigured, and the fact that I felt the abnormalities dragged my spirit; whenever I was alone, I would cry my eyes out and stare at my reflection in the mirror in horror. Upon closer inspection, the disease began to take an apparent toll, and its symptoms spread superficially and mentally as the lesions were populating. I thought that I was ugly and disfigured. My body grew weak and became stale. I noticeably saw a drooping on the right side of my face (which is Bell's palsy). It appeared mild. At first, I thought my mind was playing tricks on me, but within the final days of summer, I began to see what the other people around me noticed. My face looked as if Picasso had painted me himself. However, I was far from a work of art.

I began to have speech paralysis, where my speech became slurred, my tongue became heavy, and it was practically impossible for people to understand me. I almost swallowed my tongue ever since public speaking was traumatizing.

When high school began, I was repulsed by the sight of my face. My nerves impeded everything I tried to do. I constantly felt humiliated and scrutinized by my peers. The humiliation crumbled my self-esteem. MS kept me self-conscious and uncomfortable for years, forcing me into dark places mentally and emotionally. I felt awkward about my appearance because my motor and cognitive skills weren't functioning normally, and I thought it; others could also see it. I began to have indifference towards my parents for enrolling me into a Private Cath-olic school, as well as hatred and jealousy toward the students there. I was teased and provoked often. Especially from the continuous weight gain and bruises that MS left me with. That was just the beginning of the bullying I went through. I couldn't understand why my parents would enroll me in a place so far and different from what I was used to —mainly because I was so sick. I should be closer to home encase of an emergency. I also thought they shouldn't waste their money on private education for me, especially if –as I felt at the time – I was going to die anyway. My older siblings went to our hometown's public school, within walking distance of our home. My private school was forty-five minutes to an hour away.

When my mother submitted my application for the private school, it was the fall of fifth grade, and I had no idea she was scouting schools for me. That spring, I had taken my entrance exam with hundreds of other kids, which I winged, yet I still got in. I wanted to fail because I figured I could go to public school in my hometown and follow in my brother and sister's footsteps if I didn't pass. It was bound to happen. The pressure was intense and active since her mind was made up. My argument was, *"why me?"*; if Stephanie and Sacha went to public school, why should I be forced to attend one of the top seven private schools? I felt immense pressure to live up to whom my mother thought I could be.

My aunt had placed her daughter in the same prestigious institu-tion and got expelled. Not to mention she was able. My neighbors' children were currently in attendance there are well. What made me so different? After my mother spoke to their parents, her mind was made up. It was a definite sacrifice she wanted to make for me. I saw it as punishment. I never had the option to say no. I often thought, *how can I compare to healthy kids?* They had nothing stopping them from attaining their excellence, and I have an enormous monster between me and mine.

I wished I could go back and retake my admissions test. Before my acceptance, my mother often criticized and talked about her disappointment if I couldn't get into school because I was sick. My family recanted, day in and day out, about how I wouldn't pass the exam. It was almost a nightly dinner conversation as I felt the pressure of trying to prove to my family that I was intelligent and not broken. I would have to suffer and become a disappointment, but to her amazement and my distress, I was accepted. My mother already held such high standards for her children, and there was no exception for my pain. Once I came home a received that acceptance letter, her average for me rose even higher. I anxiously did as well. I couldn't afford what she needed to see from me. My mother wasn't the type to ever give up on her investments. She centered her energy, money, and time around my health but not so much on my wellness.

When I arrived at the hospital, my moment of freedom was extracted from me when lying there, staring me in the face, was my acceptance letter from the esteemed school of my mother's choice. My mother didn't want to open the package. She wanted me to hold her accountable for whatever the verdict was. The envelope lay there the rest of the summer unmoved under the pile of mail waiting for me. Once she opened it, she was so proud of me that he began to tell the world.

The embarrassment of getting into a prestigious school made me feel like part of a sideshow in the circus. My acceptance wasn't an honor for me; I felt cursed. Already instilled in my head, I knew I wouldn't be able to make it through a week of Private Catholic school or any school for that fact under my current circumstances. Half my body was going in and out of numbness, and I was also drooling out the side of my face. The fatigue threw my sleep pattern into a whirlwind daze. I would try to stay awake for school, but I would get most of my sleep during the day; I became a complete insomniac. I lay wide awake, praying for rest to hide from searing migraines, facial paralysis, and twitching.

My hemifacial spasms were in full swing. As I began to walk to the bus stop in the late cold winter months, my face convulsed and spasmed randomly like a beating drum, and my eyelid, my lips, and the entire right side of my face had a pulse of their own. The dysfunctionality of my body inhibited my spirit. The sensation was replaced with a weakness, numb gnawing, and slow reflexes filled with sharp pins and needles that ran up and down my face, legs, and arms on both sides of my body. I felt a similar sensation before I left the hospital that summer but not as intense. From brutality, the extremes of hot to cold, no matter the temperature, I would experience constant pain.

The doctors gave me some anti-viral and anti-seizure medications, which came with side effects, including nausea, colds, vomiting, and depression. I began to envision and believe that people could see all my endless imperfections in real time. The only things that helped call me were Mammie Lea's teas and the therapy with rolling the nutmeg around in my mouth. Some of my symptoms eventually dissipated. The severe twitching wouldn't subside for almost another year. The involuntary muscle spasm took over my body, and the pricking of millions of pins and needles throughout my body left me in anguish and exhausted for about the same length of time.

I discovered that I had double vision in the hallways, walking down the street, or staring at any object. It was alarming that I would be talking and unable to keep up in class discussions or focus on the backboard or projectors. In a few instances, drool would leak out the side of my mouth from the lack of sensation in my face. Many of my issues seemed to show that I was physically handicapped, which led me to suffer from constant embarrassment and insecurities. I remember the feeling of students running down the hallways calling for help one winter morning because my body went limp, and I went into full exacerbation. I had to be rolled out into the nurse's office in a wheelchair. All I kept thinking was, why now? Why couldn't you have waited till we got home? Why would my parents leave me out to suffer through constant daily embarrassment and pain?

I had to carry around a washcloth or tissues to wipe the saliva dripping out the side of my lifeless lip. If I forgot, my mother often reminded me in the most ostentatious way possible. My face was so numb to the touch I could feel saliva oozing from my jaw. My doctors began scheduling me to start trials on new medications and discontinued steroids. It took months to get authorization from insurance to clear me. My symptoms amplified and became more prominent, like the lesions in my brain.

MRI Number 3 of 3

The feet that used to glide me across the shiny hardwood floors of my living room would lay lifeless for years. My body language was abstract, sharp, and calculated. I was trying not to be too awkward most of the time; I would imagine how I would die the other half. I resembled an alcoholic trying to maintain their footing. I became robotic. I also lost my vision as optic neuritis began to take over my sight. Optic neuritis is the inflammation of the optic nerve bundle, which can cause involuntary eye movement and pain, sensitivity to light, and loss of vision in one or both eyes. I would close one eye, trying to focus on the other. My sense of taste was also out of sorts. I tried to eat but began noticing a change in my taste buds. Everything tasted metallic. This was only year two, dealing with this diabolical undiagnosed disease, and it seemed not to be letting up.

Learning the symptoms of auto-immune diseases frustrated me. Every sign could be associated with one disease or many, and I was experiencing them all almost instantaneously. Any pressure against, obstructed, or interrupted nerve can affect how the signals from your face and brain to your toes and every other functional organ in the body can be affected. This may cause cognitive and physical difficulties or lifelong impairment. It was nothing other than my cells eating away at my nerves that wouldn't allow the impulses to move accordingly and freely. Figuring out what ailment was slowly mauling me internally was hard for doctors to understand. First, a stroker bared similarities. Although rare, thousands of people in the UK alone are diagnosed with hemifacial spasms. The University of Maryland documented that every hundred thousand men and fifteen of every thousand women get this symptom. The onset age is around forty-four years of age.

Another rare medical diagnosis affecting two hundred thousand cases annually is Bell's palsy. Anything that triggers an imbalance can lead to chronic disability for life and even death. I wasn't aware that my body was out of *its* homeostasis. My young static mind couldn't process that type of knowledge. Bits and pieces of me became impoverished as I lost faith and hope. It was a rare occurrence for MS to happen to a younger demographic as young as me, let alone my race. My age only continued to complicate and challenge the doctors. Many ongoing inconclusive tests were performed and are still used today to make an educated guess. The tests concluded that the internal chaos imaged on MRI was parallel to what was seen.

Multiple Sclerosis provoked my awkward, crooked, and gated walk. Kids made fun of my clinging to the hallway walls and lockers for dear life. It was more than just hemifacial spasms because as time continued, other symptoms accelerated. Therefore, the doctors kept raising the medication dosage without an actual diagnosis. Yet the MRIs populated white matter (scars or lesions), followed by other physical symptoms. Doctors threw out the diagnosis of Lyme disease as their most educated guess. Around 1996, Lyme was a significant disease in the black community because it was gaslighted away. It now had come to the fore-front of many black medical diagnoses. Lyme is an infectious disease spread by tick bites followed by a red rash, migraine, fever, and brain fog. Fortunately, I hadn't been anywhere woodland nor bitten by any-thing. Multiple Sclerosis share all these similar characteristics, which made that much harder to pinpoint my diagnosis. It was an intricate and exciting process of elimination that may have cost me my life and mental wellness.

When there is no apparent cause or root, the disease is idiopathic and of no known origin. The children's idiopathic illnesses are Abdominal Epilepsy, Autism, Benign Rolandic Epilepsy, Cerebral Palsy Epilepsy, and Fibromyalgia. Juvenile Myoclonic Epilepsy, Migraine, Tuberous Sclerosis Complex, and Multiple Sclerosis.

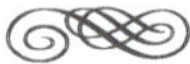

II

Dancing on Thin Ice

"The closest you can come to God is through creativity" ~Debbie Allen.

My soul danced in the twilight as doctors continued to draw blood and run tests. Regardless of how often they poked and probed me, it didn't break me because I was scared, confused, and in pain. My mind and body were on sensory overload. Pain happened in abundance, and it became my constant once it began. My spinal fluid being drawn and an exorbitant amount of bloodwork, which led to only dead ends, was the catalyst of my pain thresh hold. Each inconclusive answer opened more questions and rounds of new examinations to find a solution. The doctor compared which disease I may have by elimination, one after the other. There was no actual test, but everything was left up for further analysis because of my age, ethnicity, and symptoms. I didn't feel supported, which made it so easy for me to want to give up. I didn't understand why no one was being transparent.

MS had a way of violating me, just like the people around me more and more every day. I was bandaged in anxiety, twitching, sleep deprivation, emotional and intellectual instability, gait, and unfathomable insecurities. It all prayed heavily on my spirit. I tried to ignore the obvious, but there was no escaping it. When all seemed well, there were little reminders like tremors or the fact that my shoes would go missing every other month because my father had to take them to the shoemaker to rebuild the soles. Papa (father) knew the Russian shoemaker on a first-name basis (Michael) because of the many visits he had to make to keep my shoes from being thrown out. I would sit my penny loafers on the wooden staircase, and when they went missing, I knew they were getting repaired, or I missed placed them again. Papa would take them Friday and pick them up Sunday morning after he left the Haitian bakery. I would come in from church with Manma Lea, and they were, restored like brand new.

My balance was nonexistent on my right side. He made sure extra attention was paid to that. My gait wore my shoes and withered my soul. Sometimes Michael would have to rebuild them from scratch. Seeing it made my insecurities even more apparent. The inability not to be able to walk straight became an utter embarrassment and made me recoil and seclude myself. I often looked forward to not attending school or being pulled out of class. It was tragic that it was to go to a doctor's appointment or because I was too sick, but at times, I had to fall in line with the lesser evil.

Appointments centered around my relapses, new symptoms, and finding the best medication. Every time I had an exacerbation, my father was on standby to accompany my mother on the long drive out to the University, where my neurologist had been a resident. It was approximately two hours out on Long Island from my home. When we arrived, blood work and MRI would be done on my brain and spine (with and without contrast) individually for forty-five minutes and were done three times during my first year without a diagnosis. Although my spine never had any lesions, my mind continued that the MRIs did show several abnormalities. It has been visible for two years that my lesion began creating deep fissures in my brain and multiplying while I was actively in treatment. There was never any positivity or silver lining that followed my appointments.

The awful feeling of fire ants marching and biting up and down my legs. It was a numbing burning sensation eating at my nerves night and day. The trend began to run down my back like strobe lights flickering as I lifted and lowered my head. To *be in* my skin was uncomfortable. At times when I walked into the appointment with no sensation or symptom to mention, but as I was leaving the doctor's office, I would feel a prickling or as if I was stepping on shards of tiny glass under the sole of my feet. With every staggering gaited step, I placed pressure on the bottom of my foot and felt as if it was being lacerated from the inside out. Multiple sharp shooting pins and needles riddled my legs, preventing me from getting to my classes or finishing any task. What were these spots that were impeding my existence?

During my desperation to find a cure, I never thought my treatments would further my pain. I was under the assumption that medication was made to alleviate symptoms, but they were doing the opposite. I was never explained the risks of taking them. Therefore, I took them out of good faith because of my mother. The steroids began my introduction to many different drug trials. Steroids were my gateway drug before I knew there was such a thing; I became a prisoner to the ambiguity of my circumstances. They were trying everything to minimize or stop my pain. It took years to be still, listen to my body, and open my mind. I was so overwhelmed and angry. I was looking for anything that would change my course of pain by any means. Because of the chemical balance, this sent my mind and emotions into a whirlwind of physiological and psychological despair. I was in a daze and confused and hormonal, as my period came twice within a three-year time frame in the form of large blood clots; the doctor decided to place me on birth control, which further sent my body out of alignment. I often wondered when I would wake up from this nightmare.

It took over two years of ongoing tests and inconclusive lab results to conclude on a disease I'm still unsure about. Within three years, my parents did know what to do. My parents listened to the recommendations based on the doctor's orders. We began medication on how to treat this phantom disease but never settled. I couldn't envision a road to recovery for years. Doctor's never alluded to one. My mother's relentless search led to her becoming the number one leading physician in pediatric neurology. My mother valued anyone who knew that field of study because nothing seemed to add up. She placed much faith in science, but grandma and I weren't sold. Scared and alone, I knew that two and half years of inability to pinpoint such a disease left me almost entirely incapable of understanding how to care for myself properly. I began to feel like a zombie. No matter how much praying my grandmother did and how hard my mother worked, it couldn't take my pain away.

New symptoms rose, and my risk of relapsing and returning to the hospital increased. I couldn't focus on my health, let alone my schoolwork. I worried about never getting the chance to experience life before I died and what happened after death. I wondered how much pain would be in before id left this earth. I continued to follow doctors' orders along with their aggressive treatments. Their main concern was reducing or preventing the lesions from getting larger or multiplying. My body functions became dormant, as all I wanted to do was sleep. The idea of a new medication only brought about new symptoms, complications, and more active lesions. I had never experienced stress and anxiety of this magnitude. The only thing I could lean on was my grandmother and mother. My new standard was running tests and preparing for the massive disappointment.

I began my research seven years before covid, wondering what I was looking for. Their internet search engine wasn't the most reliable way to research and find the things I needed to know. I relied on whatever the doctors would tell me and pamphlets from the doctor's office. Thank goodness I had some scholarly bone left in my body.

According to Discovery Forum, America has one million cases and two hundred new patients diagnosed weekly. Globally, two point three million humans live with this multiple sclerosis. Eighty-five percent of people receive the initial diagnosis of relapse and remitting multiple sclerosis (RRMS). In two thousand and fifteen, Neurology Clinic Practice documented that out of sixty thousand articles published about MS, only one hundred thirteen articles cover MS in African Americans, which is less than point two percent of the articles. In a study conducted in two thousand twelve by Military Medicine, forty-six percent more cases in blacks than non – Hispanic white.

Pediatric on-set multiple Sclerosis (P.O.M.S) is also recognized as juvenile MS; according to the MS Society, it addresses POMS accrues to children between the ages of sixteen to eighteen, which only makes up ten percent of patients. Under the age of ten, only point one percent. The youngest child diagnosed on record was just two years old. I learned that my rarity must be documented to help others to help and shed light on the disease.

MS is usually considered an adult condition diagnosed in people twenty to forty years old, but MS is becoming more prevalent in young adults. Unfortunately, there isn't enough evidence gathered. Still, the most mainstream proof I've read for minority and juvenile MS is that it is way less common and improperly diagnosed and documented. Doctors also use the Evoked Potential Test. The Evoked Potential Test is a series of tests that stimulate the auditory to send signals to the nerve, leg, and arm by electronic pulse.

Both my mom and the doctor were adamant about me being on medication. Because I never met any metrics. An inflammatory drug was prescribed to keep me from exacerbations and the inflammation down, and there was no talking my mother out of it. The doctors administered steroids to me in the hopes of subduing the re-accruing symptoms and complications I was facing. Back then, that was the practical way to deal with anything disrupting the nervous system. The doctors needed a way to keep the lesions and inflammation swelling under control in my brain. Unfortunately, that wasn't enough. I was plagued with nausea, fatigue, hair loss, upset stomach, tremors, headaches and fever, welts, bruises, and scarring from puncture wounds from needles, and my menstrual cycle disappeared for months at a time.

Treatments were intense, and they changed rapidly after the first drug was approved—one after another.

Betaseron, which was my third drug by age twelve. The interferon beta-1b was used to treat not only RRMS but also Secondary Progressive disease and clinically isolated syndrome. The prescription medication was prescribed through auto-injection, and the injector's noise scared me. Therefore, I would go as my mom to give it to me when I was too anxious and my hand was shaking. My problems were often unsolved with a fear that ricocheted and may place me back in the hospital. I began to think that I had bigger things to worry about than my health. Before my diagnosis, I took three therapy treatment medications in the first two years. During that time, I relapsed many times, and without warning, the exacerbations began to lap the time I was put on this earth. There was no alleviation with the medications. I thought I was to take one pill for the rest of my life, and it was the doctor's job to find the most suitable one. This was just the beginning of my suffering. Joint pain, fever, headache, dizziness, and insomnia led to further disability and complications, which prolonged my finding any justifiable treatment that worked.

I felt like a lab rat, and all I was worthy of was trial and error—no physical therapy or psychologist. I was lost in a space that wasn't mine. Without an outlet or anyone to lead me or talk to, I began to view myself as a child unworthy of life and love. Children don't get to have an opinion, and If I had any, I wasn't given anything that had preventative measures to protect me. I had to take medicine, rather I liked it or not. I was trapped with the perception that I needed a drug to make me feel or alleviate my pain, but I didn't see any alleviation in taking them. The drugs didn't pacify nor inhibit anything; I suffered more symptoms. There was much false hope in the medication that was given to me. I was riding too high on expectations and not understanding the severity of my circumstances. I placed my hope in an industry that didn't see me. Depending on expectations only hurt me mentally and emotionally and stuck me in a rut for over a decade and a half.

I couldn't leave nor walk away from this new life. I was strung out and left in an environment with no friends and no one I could confine because no one understood. It was just my thoughts and I because I couldn't believe it. I became more withdrawn and isolated from doctors' appointments. I had been humiliated at school and ashamed of what had become of me in such a short time; negative thoughts plagued me every waking minute of the day.

I always wished I would find a way to remove all this pain. A cure or a calm end to it all. No one understood the impact MS was having on me; therefore, I began to think I needed to step up and do something I may regret. The pain I was feeling was overwhelming, and taking matters into my own hands was inevitable. No one could feel or see my decomposition and not understand the disconnect. My mother was so focused on trusting the science t she acted as if the doctors and their medicine had a cure. My grandmother's appeasement and coddling gave me a sense of calm. Father was barely there, working himself to exhaustion. My siblings were far too busy to tend to me. Sometimes I felt that my life was suspended in time, just me there dangling with my toes sweeping the floor as I took my last breath. I could never have found enough empathy or support in my family and within myself. I was slowly losing my sanity day by day with every waking breath.

Multiple Sclerosis was one of the last conclusions the doctors would have conjured. Finding a diagnosis and learning there was no way to fundamentally cure it made my support system even more critical in my journey—some of the most dedicated people I can never repay. The lessons you have taught are embedded in these pages. It was very stressful and frustrating for all parties involved, but they did a hell of a job keeping a brave face and me alive. Everyone deals with traumas in various ways. I gave up on myself several times before even writing a sentence in this book. Then I realized I am just one of the few who placed God and time at the front of my battle and used time and God's grace to my advantage.

12

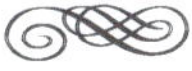

The Crucifixion

"The closest you can come to God is through creativity" ~Debbie Allen.

My soul danced in the twilight as doctors continued to test after test. They couldn't break my soul regardless of how much they continued to poke and probe me. They drew and took my spinal fluid and blood work, which, after analyzing, led to dead ends. Each inconclusive answer opened my questions and rounds of new examinations to try to find the answer. The doctor compared which disease I may have by elimination, one after the other. There was no actual test, but everything was left up for further analysis because of my age, ethnicity, and symptoms. I didn't feel supported; that is what made it so easy for me to want to give up.

MS had a way of violating me more and more every day. I was bandaged in anxiety, twitching, sleep deprivation, emotional and intellectual instability, gait, and imbalance with my walking. It all prayed on my young spirit. I had to learn how to walk all over again. My father would constantly take my shoes to the shoemaker every two to three months to rebuild the soles and heels of my penny loafers. I would sit my penny loafers on the wooden staircase where he would take them, and within a weekend, they would be restored like brand new. He would drop off my penny loafers every other month for shoe polish and fix the ran-down heel of my left foot. My balance was almost not existent. I placed much of my weight on one right side, which wore me down, often because of my gait and foot-dragging. Papa (father) knew the Russian shoemaker on a first-name basis because of the many visits he had to make to keep my loafers together.

My many doctor's visit appointments were centered around my re-lapses, new symptoms, and finding new medication. Every time I had an exacerbation, my father was on standby to accompany my mother on the long drive out to the University, where my neurologist was a resident. I was approximately two hours out on Long Island. When we arrived, blood work and MRI would be done on my brain and spine (with and without contrast) individually for forty-five minutes and were done three times during my first year without a diagnosis. Although my spine never had any lesions, my mind continued that the MRIs did show abnormalities in my brain matter and unction. It was undeniable for two years that my lesion began creating deep fissures in my brain and multiplying while I was actively on treatment. There was never any positivity or silver lining that followed my appointments.

The awful feeling of fire ants marching and biting up and down my legs. It was a numbing burning sensation eating at my nerves night and day. The trend began to run down my back like strobe lights flickering as I lifted and lowered my head. To *be in* my skin was uncomfortable. At times when I walked into the appointment with no sensation or symptom to mention, but as I was leaving the doctor's office, I would feel a prickling or as if I was stepping on shards of tiny glass under the sole of my feet. With every staggering gaited step, I placed pressure on the bottom of my foot and felt as if it was being lacerated from the inside out. Multiple sharp shooting pins and needles riddled my legs, preventing me from getting to my classes or finishing any task. What were these spots that were impeding my existence?

During my desperation, I never thought my treatments would further my pain. I was under the assumption that medication was made to alleviate symptoms, but they were doing the opposite. I was never explained the risks of taking them. Therefore, I took them out of good faith because of my mother. The steroids began my introduction to many different drug trials. Steroids were my gateway drug before I knew there was such a thing; I became a prisoner to the ambiguity of my circumstances. They were trying everything to minimize or stop my pain. It took years to be still, listen to my body, and open my mind. I was so overwhelmed and angry. I was looking for anything that would change my course of pain by any means. Because of the chemical balance, this sent my mind and emotions into a whirlwind of physiological and psychological despair. I was in a daze and confused and hormonal as my period came twice within a three-year time frame in the form of large blood clots; the doctor decided to place me on birth control, which further sent my body out of alignment. I often wondered when I would wake up from this nightmare.

Multiple Sclerosis was one of the last conclusions the doctors would have conjured. Finding a diagnosis and learning there was no way to fundamentally cure it made my support system some of the most dedicated people I can ever repay. I gave up on myself several times before even writing a chapter of this book. It was very stressful and frustrating for all parties involved, but they did a hell of a job keeping a brave face and me alive. Everyone deals with traumas in various ways. I am just one of the few who placed God and time at the front of my battle and used time and God's grace to my advantage.

It took over two years of ongoing tests and inconclusive lab results to conclude on a disease I'm still unsure about. Within three years, my parents did know what to do. My parents listened to the recommendations based on the doctor's orders. We began medication on how to treat this phantom disease but never settled. I couldn't envision a road to recovery for years. Doctor's never alluded to one. My mother's relentless search led to the number one leading physician in pediatric neurology. My mother valued anyone who knew that field of study because nothing seemed to add up. She placed much faith in science, but grandma and I weren't sold. Scared and alone, I knew that two and half years of inability to pinpoint such a disease left me almost entirely incapable of understanding how to care for myself properly. I began to feel like a zombie. No matter how much praying my grandmother did and how hard my mother worked, it couldn't take my pain away.

New symptoms rose, and my risk of relapsing and returning to the hospital increased. I couldn't focus on my health, let alone my schoolwork. I worried about never getting the chance to experience life before I died and what happened after death. I wondered how much pain would be in before id left this earth. I continued to follow doctors' orders along with their aggressive treatments. Their main concern was reducing or preventing the lesions from getting larger or multiplying. My body functions became dormant, and so did the world, yet with the new change in medication, they continue to get larger. I had never experienced stress and anxiety of this magnitude. The only thing I could lean on was my grandmother and mother. My new standard was running tests and preparing for the massive disappointment.

I began my research seven years before covid, not knowing what I was looking for. There internet search engine wasn't the most reliable way to research and find the things I needed to know. I relied on whatever the doctors would tell me and pamphlets from the doctor's office. Thank goodness I had some scholarly bone left in my body.

According to Discovery Forum, America has one million cases and two hundred new patients diagnosed weekly. Globally, two point three million humans live with this multiple sclerosis. Eighty-five percent of people receive the initial diagnosis of relapse and remitting multiple sclerosis (RRMS). In two thousand and fifteen, Neurology Clinic Practice documented that out of sixty thousand articles published about MS, only one hundred thirteen articles cover MS in African Americans, which is less than point two percent of the articles. In a study conducted in two thousand twelve by Military Medicine, forty-six percent more cases in blacks than non – Hispanic white.

Pediatric on-set multiple Sclerosis (P.O.M.S) is also recognized as juvenile MS; according to the MS Society, it addresses POMS accrues to children the ages sixteen to eighteen, which only makes up ten percent of patients. Under the age of ten, only point one percent. The youngest child diagnosed on record was just two years old. I learned that my rarity must be documented to help others.

MS is usually considered an adult condition diagnosed in people twenty to forty years ago, but MS is becoming more prevalent in young adults. Unfortunately, there isn't enough evidence gathered. Still, the most mainstream proof I've read for minority and juvenile MS is that it is way less common and improperly diagnosed and documented. Doctors also use the Evoked Potential Test. The Evoked Potential Test is a series of tests that stimulate the auditory to send signals to the nerve, leg, and arm by electronic pulse. Both my mom and the doctor were adamant about me being on medication. Because I never met any metrics. An inflammatory drug was prescribed to keep me from exacerbations and the inflammation down, and there was no talking my mother out of it. The doctors administered steroids to me in the hopes of subduing the re-accruing symptoms and complications I was facing. Back then, that was the practical way to deal with anything disrupting the nervous system. The doctors needed a way to keep the lesions and inflammation swelling under control in my brain. Unfortunately, that wasn't enough. I was plagued with nausea, fatigue, hair loss, upset stomach, tremors, headaches and fever, welts, bruises, and scarring from puncture wounds from needles, and my menstrual cycle disappeared for months at a time. Treatments were intense, and they changed rapidly after the first drug was approved—one after another.

Betaseron, which was my third drug by age twelve. The interferon beta-1b was used to treat not only RRMS but also Secondary Progressive disease and clinically isolated syndrome. The prescription medication was prescribed through auto-injection, and the injector's noise scared me. Therefore, I would go as my mom to give it to me when I was too anxious, and my hand wasn't steady enough. My problems were often unsolved with a fear that ricocheted and may place me back in the hospital. I began to think that I had bigger things to worry about than my health. Before my diagnosis, I took three therapy treatment medications in the first two years. During that time, I relapsed many times, and without warning, the exacerbations began to lap the time I was put on this earth. There was no alleviation with the medications. I thought I was to take one pill for the rest of my life, and it was the doctor's job to find the most suitable one. This was just the beginning of my suffering. Joint pain, fever, headache, dizziness, and insomnia led to further disability and complications, which prolonged my finding any justifiable treatment that worked.

I felt like a lab rat, and all I was worthy of was trial and error—no physical therapy or psychologist. I was lost in a space that wasn't mine. Without an outlet or anyone to lead me or talk to, I began to view myself as a child unworthy of life and love. Children don't get to have an opinion, and If I had any, I wasn't given anything that had preventative measures to protect me. I had to take medicine, rather I liked it or not. I was trapped with the perception that I needed a drug to make me feel or alleviate my pain, but I didn't see any positivity in them. The drugs didn't pacify nor inhibit anything; I suffered more symptoms. There was much false hope in the medication that was given to me. I was riding too high on expectations and not understanding the severity of what I was living. I placed my hope into the drug industry, which only hurt me mentally and emotionally and stuck me in a rut for over a decade and a half.

I couldn't leave nor walk away from this new life. I was strung out and left in an environment with no friends and no one I could confine. It was just my thoughts and I because I couldn't believe it. I became more withdrawn and isolated from doctors' appointments. I had been humiliated at school and ashamed of what had become of me in such a short time; negative thoughts plagued me every waking minute of the day.

I always wished I would find a way to remove all this pain. A cure or a calm end to it all. No one understood the impact MS was having on me; therefore, I began to think I needed to step up and do something I may regret. The pain I was feeling was overwhelming, and taking matters into my own hands was inevitable. No one could feel or see my decomposition and not understand the disconnect. My mother was so focused on me not being sick that she acted as if she overlooked the fact that I was hurting. My grandmother's appeasement and coddling gave me a sense of calm. Father was barely there, working himself to exhaustion. My siblings were far too busy to tend to me. Sometimes I felt that my life was suspended in time, just me there dangling. I could never have found enough empathy or support in my family and within myself. I was slowly losing my sanity day by day with every waking breath.

13

Trial and Error

"Drugs: Compounds that block a step in your biological pathways. Vegetables: Compounds that restore steps in your biochemical pathways, restoring health."- Dr. Terry Wahls

I got on the yellow neon-colored school bus and sat at the back. It was a quiet afternoon on the school bus because many students were in extracurricular activities; all the bullies were busy with practice. My eyes began to feel heavy like cinder blocks. I had some quiet before my long evening began. When I experienced days like this, I loved them because I looked forward to the hour-long bus ride filled with peace, no gossip or bother. My only wish would have been longer bus rides like this so I could have rested more. There was always a certain feeling of comfort I got from a moving vessel that always put me at ease. I would curl up in a ball and rest my head on my bookbag. After the hour ride, I heard the breaks of the school bus screech to a halt. Interrupted, I jumped up, popped my head up, and peered my weary eyes out the window.

"Wait! Hold on; I'm getting off," I yawned at the bus driver as I grabbed my book bag and blazer. I leaped up as quickly as possible. Holding on to the back of the chairs, I quickly stumbled to the front towards the exit. I took two steps off the bus and completely missed the final stair, or my legs stopped working again. I fell flat on my face onto the hot concrete. The bus driver unfastened his seat belt and jumped off the bus to pick me up. He asked me if I was okay. I got up and told him to leave me alone and that I was *good.*

I dusted the gravel off my school uniform, grabbed my book bag and blazer, and shuffled off, dragging my pride behind me. I squinted down the block to measure the distance to the corner. My vision was stormy and blurry. My eyes were hurting but walks with my grandmother allowed me to navigate when I was symptomatic quickly. My right eye began to flutter and twitch without missing a beat.

"I just want to lie down," I mumbled. "One two, one two, " I chanted, trying to tightrope my way home. I wiped my eye as if that would make the twitching subside, but my vision started to flutter more vigorously as if those nerves had a mind of their own. I tried to focus on the sidewalk but saw two of everything. My legs trembled as I pushed through my gait, and I continued to navigate my way home. My goal was to make it home so I wouldn't collapse again in the streets. I was afraid that the next time I wouldn't be able to get up.

I finally arrived home and approached the side door that my mother had left ajar during warmer months. We enjoyed the ventilation, which would flow through the kitchen into our home. My mother heard the shuffling of the worn-out soles of my black penny loafers. It hadn't even been three months since they were replaced. I walked into my kitchen past my mother, trying not to draw attention to my gait. My right side was weaker than my left, which kept my walk very deliberate. I often spoke to myself, searching for encouragement, muttering the words my mother and grandmother often told me.

"There you go, you got it, one... two... one... two." Exhausted, one loafer at a time, I swept the ceramic kitchen floor as I walked past my mother while she was brewing tea. I shuffled past her with a quick hello and

waved it, hoping she wouldn't stop and ask me how I was feeling or diagnose my mood, which she was great at. I tossed my bag, as usual, on the dining room table. She turned, and in the same instance, she noticed I looked visibly upset through my facial twitching, which was more bothersome and uncomfortable than anything.

I asked my mother where Mammie Lea was. She told me she went to the grocery store. I was left with the one person I didn't want around me when I felt unwell. She could nit-pick and nag me to death. I sat on the bar stool at the kitchen peninsula and cradled my head with my hands. My mother never asked me how I was feeling. Yet, she automatically assumed I had an issue. She walked to the kitchen cabinet, grabbed a jar filled with large nutmegs, washed it off, and placed one in a napkin before me. I knew I was to put it in my mouth. My mom and grandmother knew the medicinal and therapeutic properties would help tame my facial spasms and change the contour of my mouth from the Bell's Palsy. She asked me if I had drunk enough water for the day. I guess that was her way of assessing how unwell I was feeling. I lifted my head and gave her a brief nod. My mother placed a cup of water in front of me as well. She ordered me to drink the water and put the nutmeg in my mouth. Hydration was the least of my worries. My mouth drooped to the right side of my face, and my speech slurred.

I looked like my face was melting with my facial spasms and muscle contortions in full effect. I sat impatiently in the dining room while my mother stood across from me in the kitchen. I could feel her eyes peering over her shoulder. Our kitchen was divided from the dining room by a peninsula. I was trying to regain the energy to hurry off to my room. I was to carry on as if my inevitable self-destruction was normal. I wanted to be alone.

Before I went to my room, I asked my mother a few questions. Talking to my mother was like talking to an optimistic realist. Her reality didn't site my understanding. I thought she disliked me because of how calmly she acted toward my frustrations and apprehensions. She gave me options when I needed guidance and direction when I needed concise answers. I understand the frustration with what she knew. She was trying to do her best as a pre-teen mommy with an undiagnosed chronic autoimmune deficiency that she had never heard of. Still, I was so annoyed by her as she scrutinized my every move; unknowingly, she was helping me build my character. She always told me the truth and was very direct. That intimidated me when I was younger, but now, I look up to her frankness and appreciate it. When I was in pain, she would advocate," *if something hurts you, hurt it back,*" and *"the impossible was only impossible if I thought it was impossible."* Her stern and transparent rhetoric was off-putting and only continued to make me feel more alienated. She held me to a certain standard, which was much pressure. She told me that life would never be easy for me. I shouldn't expect rules to change just because I was an unwell child. She wouldn't show me any leniency, nor did she have any to spare. Mommy Fanny held me accountable for all my good and evil actions since my brother did most of the reporting. She was an immigrant, so I knew her logic was deeply rooted. I didn't care to explore the intricacies of her philosophy because I didn't find any relevance. Later in life, I realized it was the most real logic.

My mind was currently learning how to make itself up and was occupied with the spasticity of my body. I touched the surface of my face and felt worms scouring my flesh's interior walls. I even forgot the questions I had asked her. Everything becomes less relevant you're dealing with intense pain. The feeling of pins and needles attacking my legs, face, and arms was overwhelming. I hated it there, inside my body. These sensations and all this conversation aggravated my soul. The pressure was too much for me to bare. I broke the conversation and told her I was going to my room, yet she continued the conversation as if whatever I said had no bearing. I knew she would never see my side. I couldn't see hers beyond my pre-pubescent angst or irrational mood swings. I became increasingly upset as my mother tried to calm me down and change my mind. She insisted that I was too excited and needed to relax. The worst thing you can tell a person with chronic anxiety is to relax. My mom walked to the fridge and poured me fresh water. I drank the water and tried to get up. When I went to rise from the bar stool, I lost my balance and plopped back down into my chair. Then I slowly lowered myself back down to the dining room chairs. My face began to feel fuzzy, tingling to the point that it turned numb.

I usually felt this during an exacerbation. I held my face and felt the twitching that ran relentlessly through my eyelids, making my lips and nostrils quiver. I was infuriated by the anguish of listening to my mother inconsiderate of my frustrations. She had no idea what was happening inside of me. My body made me conform to a new normal, trying to resist the pain, which was my master manipulator. Another dead-ended argument that prayed on whatever nerve I had left. My pleading with my mother never got me far. She handed me a teacup and a napkin. I was drooling out the side of my mouth again.

I begged my parents every day to withdraw me from private school and place me in public school. I further reasoned with her that she was wasting money on education I found no value in, nor would they ever see the fruits of their labor. I couldn't concentrate, which made me feel dunce. My brain filled with lesions only hindered my concentration and cut short my attention span to comprehend all lesson plans. She told me that if I weren't so wrapped up in trying to join academic and sports clubs and tried to focus more on my scholastics, I would do better with my studies. For God's sake, I was failing gym and only doing well in music. After trying to rationalize with her, she would send me to my room, and I cried and slept off the frustration but not the symptoms. If my mother was doing her best, why would she allow me to struggle and risk wasting so much money investing in education? Even my neurologist told me that I might never see graduation. I felt she didn't care to see things from my perspective. I could barely wake up on time for school or remember my class schedule. She would tell me to tape it inside every binder and notebook I used for my classes but never helped me do so. I often found myself running into the guidance counselor's office asking for a reprint of my class schedule; my memory was growing fuzzier.

Multiple Sclerosis always had a way of making me second guess my worth. MS blew up my inabilities and insecurities in massive proportions. It challenged my assertiveness, and I continued to think my gut instincts second. Twenty minutes or so passed after failing to prove my point, and I finally gave up and went to my room and slammed the door behind me.

I was angry, disturbed, and unwilling to understand why it was so hard for my mother to comprehend me. I felt like I'd always received the stick's short end. I grew bitter and resentful toward her. There were no shortcuts for me. I became unapologetic and brazen during our conversations. When we spoke, my tongue became serrated, short, and bold. I resented her because she wouldn't allow me to be an average child. In all reality, it was MS that stifled my growth. She wanted me to reach her standards without letting me cut corners. She required me to do well in school. My parents were already spending thousands of dollars on my education. I often feared getting summer school because summer courses would have cost upwards of three hundred dollars per class per week.

I had to be the first of my siblings to be home and the first to go to bed (not by choice, most of the time). I couldn't keep up with the basic adolescent regime. I was drowning.

My days were mundanely filled with solitude and pessimism. I drifted between complacency and the heavy burden of anxiety. I searched for a way through my circumstances. I hadn't understood that my attitude and mindset would affect my life's trajectory. I was outraged and uncomfortable.

I walked into the bathroom and washed my face. Staring at my reflection was sheer torture. I squinted my eyes and watched as my face danced buoyantly in the mirror. My review looked repulsive. I grew frustrated and bawled up my fist to punch myself in the eye, hoping the twitching would stop. Then again and again and again and again. I cried and heaved into a washed rag, muffling my tears which just caused my face to convulse even more. I ran into my room and continued crying until I passed out.

My mother called for me. She walked up the stairs to my room, made her way in without knocking, and found me fast asleep. She nudged me to wake up, but I didn't want to leave my bed. She told me that I was knocked out cold. My mother shook and startled me out of my deep slumber, which I'd been sleeping for three hours. I woke up and felt like a measly ten minutes had passed. The sleep interruption made me more anxious, although the twitching dulled for the moment. She gingerly helped me up and got me dressed. When I got to the den and was seated, the doorbell rang. My heart began racing as my mother went to answer it.

Today was the day I had my first at-home infusion for a new trial drug prescribed by my former neurologist. Stabilizing my symptoms was the objective because it sure wasn't to find a cure. I'm pretty sure I was a particular case. In anticipation, my anxiety went through the roof. I heard chatter and footsteps approaching the family room, where I waited impatiently. The nurse stepped into the room and greeted me. She asked me several questions and told me what to expect from that day's procedure. She asked me about my sleeping patterns, bowel movements, and last menstrual cycle, which had gone missing since its first appearance last summer. She asked me if I had any other symptoms." I replied no because I wanted this day to be over with.

I nodded and prepared myself for the disclosers and warning about the medication and procedure as the nurse listed the many mishaps that could occur. I listened as she took her notations. My mother would step in from time to time when I didn't understand and answer on my behalf shortly after the nurse put her notepad down and began to set up her equipment. As I braced for my first-ever at-home infusion, my tummy turned in knots. She had my mother fill out and sign some legal waivers and forms. She took my temperature and blood pressure. She pulled out a few syringes, alcohol pads, and IV medicine bags and laid them neatly on the table. I asked her if it was going to hurt. She said, "No', but her hesitation led me to believe it was a lie. I waited for her to tell me that this medication would cure me. As she put the needle in my arm, I winced, and I still do now, even though I know exactly how much pain to expect.

I quickly became uninterested when it came to her reasoning for the

IV. I began to focus on the bitter yet familiar weird metallic taste it left in my mouth. The nurse told me that the iron rust taste in my mouth was typical. I immediately ask my mother for the juice to coat the taste. She ran into the kitchen. When she returned with the liquid, the nurse set up another fluid bag, which she explained to me was penicillin. I asked her if that would leave a taste. She told me it wouldn't. As I expected, that, too, was a lie. Suddenly, my pulse began to race, and my skin began to itch.

The nurse asked me how I was feeling. I automatically responded that I was okay. Then she started the intravenous steroid drip. I felt my eyes continue to well up, my mouth felt dry, my palms felt cold and clammy, and I felt warm. In mid-conversation, they both stopped and looked over at me. I asked my mother if she saw something on my cheek, as I felt like something bit me. I touched my face, and I had welts. The nurse checked my chest and arms; there were welts there too. Then she took my temperature. Quickly, she stopped the infusion. I was allergic to not only penicillin but the drug that was being administered to me. Mother told me later that my temperature had risen to 106 degrees Fahrenheit. I never made it back to school for the next two weeks because I was being held under observation. I learned that day that I was allergic to penicillin and ruled out the medication.

14

Asleep

Rather than researching and assessing the underlining circumstances behind the disease and opting to move forward with the cases, the lesser happened. I listened to whatever the doctors conjured up without doing my research. Other than because I was in my mother's direct care, I didn't see another choice. The internet was not as easily accessible back then as it is now, and it wasn't easy for me to get the quality of information I needed and deserved. My mind was incapable of understanding what was at stake. The concept of being that sickly so young went over my head. I was too young and weak to explore my circumstances, rendering me helpless and hopeless. I was at the beck and call of the neurologist. Therefore, adolescence was far from nostalgic. I think about my childhood and the things I could have changed or become more aware of. My journey to diagnosis was gaslighted by the

"

uncertainties of a narrative that never allowed the time, thought, or space to be captured.

Multiple Sclerosis consumed my very being of me. I remained hostage and disheartened for the next fifteen years. My approach to handling the disease was circumstantial and pivoted based on many different emotional and pain levels. One day I would be happy, then the next day, I would be completely and utterly destructive, depressed, and in despair. Having to cope with Multiple Sclerosis while transitioning from a child to teenager was accompanied by much gray matter and hard times. Severe anxiety and stress led to early chronic depression and aggression; I had so much hate beyond dealing with the pre-pubescent precarious mood swings and environmental changes. I also faced the hurdle of bridging a transitional social gap from elementary to high school. My circumstances were unforgiving. I was shifting to a level that didn't allow my mind to grow or move on. I had no valid concept of what I was feeling. I just remembered that it had to be done by any means necessary. When I was finally diagnosed with a disease, I refused to give Multiple Sclerosis the respect it deserved. At least given a title to my symptoms.

There was no cure, and that was a hard pill to swallow. It angered and hurt me. Harsher realities, growing pains, struggles, and lack of ambition hovered over my life for many years. I suffered with my scholastics and social skills. I became the ideal extreme pessimist and introvert. My moods and habits became uncertain, awkward, and volatile. My life grew in conflict and completely unforgiving circumstances, tearing my morals.

MS moved quickly, fast, and came in waves; I rebuilt my broken spirit with the help of my grandmother and mother, working out, meditating, and learning alternative healthier habits for fueling and nourishing my body. First, I had to come to an awakening state of mind which took over a decade to surface. I did much soul-searching during the most trying times of my life, which became evident in my self-love and gratitude to my mother and ancestors. Patience and discipline became critical factors in my growth and wellness. My strength was rooted in my faith in God. Even with my faith, I was. Still, I was feeble and naïve enough to lose sight of it. I thought my world to be had been taken away from me to see the rawness of life. The life I had become accustomed to was beautiful but short-lived. My time was taken away from me. Not because I was a delinquent or my family fell on hard times, but because my adolescent life was chosen by millions to deal with this hardship, and I dealt with it all alone. People began to leave and move away from me, and so did my identity.

My loss of identity left me vulnerable and scared because the shock happened swiftly. Multiple Sclerosis was a threat, and no one could help me. Two decades later, I found myself in balance and alignment. It was homeostasis with my spirit and mind and the environment around me. I chose to find a way to pull myself out of the darkness and let my energy serve another purpose and not one that was fruitless. One is not focused on fear and hurt but on healing, hope, faith, wellness, and joy. A belief in self-love and the unconditional love of God and family became my mission. My mother made me a warrior, and my grandmother gave me heart. My epiphany was inevitable because of the women that raised me.

Disease changes live in epic proportions because diseases come with enormous upsets, setbacks, and price tags mentally, spiritually, emotionally, and financially. Along with that, they also come with an understanding of how severe the circumstances are. For a moment, I needed to realize that if I continued to lose myself, how it would affect the people that love me? Accommodations made from absolute selflessness and mercy, love, empathy, and trying to understand while I was too busy trying to figure out my pain, MS wouldn't allow me to be grateful. I could not reflect on the circumstances that stood in my way of seeing the bigger picture and living a better life. I was forsaken and allowed the daunting prognosis to take hold of my future. I came to terms in my own time with understanding the truth. I needed to fall on my face many times before I came to terms with my diagnosis. Over the years, I'd adjusted my mindset and honed the energy to manifest and change my prognosis rather than succumbing to whatever I was told. With the gavel being slammed, I experienced various stages, from denial to acceptance and sometimes through a tug-of-war between medication and holistic wellness.

"Not me! You must be mistaken." Everyone goes through a stage of denial when tragic events occur. The disbelief can be instant and brief or never accepted because it seems so far-fetched. I've learned that anything can happen to anyone of God's creatures and not to overlook the severity of the matter.

With no initial assessment, evidence, or clarification on identifying my problem, I concluded there wasn't one, and it must have been a mistake. Unable to understand the severity of what was going on, I was giving up. No therapies but only medication was afforded to me; therefore, I took whatever I was given. Once, I was told by the neurologist that there was no cure; I thought that I was at rock bottom. I began spiraling down a deep and dark place physically, mentally, and emotionally and I did even notice, nor could anyone tell. Taking that moment in and that deep breath and tackling it head-on at face value would have been most strategic, but to a nine-and-a-half-year-old, there was no strategy, just me trying to reason with my inner child and God. I didn't know there was no reason for sickness, disease, or death. I became very selfish and was only worried about how much time I didn't think I had left to live. I was caught. I'm a dangerous web, and it spun out of control. I was dealing with multitudes of mental and physical handicaps that I couldn't comprehend. Drawing my conclusions from what doctors told me when they, as medical professionals, didn't know much better themselves. My spirit imploded, and my mind and body impaled; I couldn't defy the odds because I couldn't identify my problem. I didn't believe I had an issue, but I felt every pain.

Blame: I wanted to know who did this. I most certainly wasn't going to blame myself. I was rattling my brain and trying to make sense of what was happening. I couldn't have done this to myself. I tried to place the burden and responsibility on my mother. Therefore, I began playing "the blame game." I needed to put my burden and pain on someone other than myself. I figured when I found the cause, I would be able to tell the doctors, and they could presumably give me the cure. I prayed to find anything to hold me accountable for my anguish. I believed the doctors and my family were failing me. I looked toward my friends and romantic relationships for alleviation. Still, there wasn't anything in the world that anyone could do because I had to find the strength and knowledge within myself to begin my healing journey. I started to alienate myself to avoid embarrassment and ridicule but in high school seemed as if I was a magnet. In my heart, I thought that if people weren't trying to help me, they were most certainly out to hurt me. I needed to discover who I was. As a result, I thought that God hated me or that my parents had failed me, and finally, in my later years, I began to hold myself accountable.

No one understood me. I felt that way for years because I felt so alone. My family members were less sensitive regarding my emotional and mental state. It was an approach outside of what the doctors told them. It was just a list of inabilities and symptoms after symptoms. I had to play pretend more now than ever before. If I let the kids know how weak I was at school, they would ruin me. I wore a façade for more than half my life. Inside, I was looking for support, yet I had an excellent way of brushing things off and hiding my pain. How can anyone relate to someone with a disease that no one can understand?

I had to learn how to cope. The endurance I maintained through such a hypersensitive time in my life proved that I was built to last and share my story in hopes of shedding light on such a topic as Multiple Sclerosis, mental illness, and wellness which can attack at any age.

Through this dark and daunting twilight, navigating through the shadows, I have detailed accounts of my life with Multiple Sclerosis from the beginning with diagnosis and continuing through the prognosis where I found grief. I couldn't imagine a life without my plus one (MS). Relying on scientific evidence and trial and error, my lack of transparency superseded any x-ray I ever took, and even with the ongoing counseling of my grandmother and mother, I had to liberate myself from the white, opaque hospital walls allowing my mind and heart to remained captured in for over a decade and a half.

15

Post-impressionism

Chapter 15
Post-impressionism

"There is beauty in the unfocused perspective. Once you balance your energy, a beam of light will appear from within you, filled with colors that will guide you and naturally pave your path. Follow your heart." – DLM.

Recounting my journey has taken me back through every relapse and every remission and fueled my life with moments of pride, pain, and resilience that were forced upon me. Hopefully, in my catharsis, many will find peace and know they aren't alone. Give yourself the will never to give up and some guidance. I hope to bring humanity closer to loving our individuality and the similarities using the words between these pages. I believe that a chance for change is on our horizon. No matter how hard things seem, I know the strength in my faith guided me; I hope readers can identify the same. Our choices today control our future, but what we believe determines our reality.

The human body is ridiculously more resilient than we think. The human mind is very malleable. Not everyone identifies with Multiple Sclerosis nor exhibits many of the same symptoms. Still, I know the struggles I'm sharing may help someone who could be dealing with their ailment or difficulties. I intend to spread awareness to promote positive change in society, aiding in research surrounding MS as the number of people diagnosed with MS continuously rises. I stand firm in my knowledge that there is more we can do to help in research, especially with Multiple pediatric Sclerosis, as well as any other immune diseases. No one should feel alienated or alone in their journey during their growth and self-discovery, nor do they deserve to be afraid. Humanity needs to relearn how to love and refrain from esterification a systemizing. To identify with each other, using faith, hope, kindness, respect, and reverence for all. It is imperative to be mindful and to spread the wealth of knowledge to help one another. I believe that it is more important to be heard rather than seen. We can provide a beacon of mental and emotional support for others along their journeys with any disease. It amazes me how much we can learn from one another if we listen.

Beginnings of My Carpe Diem

When the doctors were finally on the brink of my diagnosis, I was eleven years of age. I was in my final year of being a Latin schooler. Catholic School terminology for middle school and learning a dead (ancient) language in the eighth grade. Moving on, my daily life caused me immense anxiety and depression; angry, sad, resentful, bullied and lost. Beyond age eleven, I went through several stages. The last stage that signified I was ready to tackle MS was acceptance.

With tons of research, family history, self-wellness, and self-discovery, it was as if a light bulb went on and off, then back on. It gave me many intricate and valuable pieces to the puzzle in the form of questions and experiences. I was the most critical of my self-evaluation and how much I valued my life. I had to be open enough to let change happen. I could mentally, physically, spiritually, and emotionally rehabilitate myself with much physical, mental, and spiritual work.

I realized my health would never change unless I kept an open mind and heart to push through my diagnosis. I drew my focus from my grandmother's love and resilience and my mother's belief in me. They became the battery built over time in my back. I began to harness the strength to take accountability for my health. My sole responsibility was to reach past the limits set for me after a decade and a half of running away from myself and my health. I had to find a way to prioritize where my disease and my diagnosis stood in my life. To do so, I broke the rules and the standards my mother had set for me. I got into relationships that help little to no value to appease my pain and feed my ego, which we toxic to everyone involved. I shook bridges, walked across them, and began setting a standard for myself. I challenged the doctors' protocols because I never got any answers or results from treatments; therefore, I slowly began to take my health into my own hands. I adhered to everything my Mammie Lea prayed for, but I wasn't ready to be open to learning. Losing my faith as an adolescent made it hard to find it again.

My love for my grandmother fostered my relationship with God and my faith. My mother taught me that I was strong enough to persevere through anything Multiple Sclerosis could dish out. I needed to learn how to gather that energy, utilize it with reverence, focus, and love, and not only put on a face to brace for such a cold world with resilience but to go toe to toe with Multiple Sclerosis. My grandmother and mother kept me afloat no matter how sick I got with their unconditional love and devotion. My brother saved and kept me in line as my disciplinarian, but he was kind as he always referred to me as his firstborn.

Although it took me fifteen years to figure out my rhythm and balance, I only came to understand wellness and health because I had a problem and was the only person who could solve it. With the new lifestyle, I was gifted; no matter how many times Multiple Sclerosis threw me off course, relapse after relapse, flare-up after flare-up, the love of my grandmother and my mother's strength coached me back to my senses. I found greater significance in my love for myself and humanity when I focused on my wellness.

I used to blame my pain and hurt on my parents and their lack thereof awareness. Still, looking past the endless doctor appointments, needles, and relapses, I just needed a scapegoat, as this pain was too much for any child to rake on the responsibility alone. I realized my lack of knowledge only led to the manifestation of fear and relentless anxiety. I feared the unknown. I continued for years to accept more failures while maturing, learning, and enduring what was coming for me. Never again would I allow me to free-fall into despair and pity. I felt I was failing my grandmother and mother, not to mention myself. I felt as if I lacked so much of the knowledge that I deserved to be equipped to face Multiple Sclerosis and fight through my circumstances. I had to prioritize Multiple Sclerosis and where it stood in my life. Almost two decades later, I learned I had to put my life and health on a pedestal. I knew that prayers don't work if I didn't. I was finally aware that I could not structure my life around my disease and was only as boundless as my mind allowed me to be. I structured the condition around *my* life and fostered a relationship within the universe, allowing energy to flow freely and work within me. I opened my mind to options I didn't know because I was told they weren't for me.

I released my apprehension and allowed myself to open to new experiences and find concrete evidence through my experimentations to understand how this disease worked. I needed to know and understand whatever made me tick and made me tock. Granted, I was young at the time of my diagnosis, but I was still searching for where my joy went and how I could find it.

Over a decade later, I feel that being diagnosed so young silenced me enough together all my strength to combat my demons head-on. Diagnosed at a young age, I was in one steadily rising percentile. My journey will allow me to pull through some hardships and regain footing. I had ample time to grieve a lost childhood—which permitted me to attain wisdom and knowledge. I learned to build a tolerance for neurological and mental, and emotional pain and how to cope. Within those two decades, I was able to make my resiliency a lifelong battle. Whenever MS wanted to break me, I had my grandmother help me push through. As time continued, I became more in tune and invested with my body and began acknowledging the Multiple symptoms of sclerosis.

16

The Silver Lining is in Coping

"My brain cannot process failure because I have to sit there and face myself and tell myself you're a failure; I think that is almost worse than dying"- Kobe Bryant.

Tell me the whole truth and nothing but the truth. Please help me, God. Spare me the medical jargon health providers love stuffing down the patients' throats. I never wanted to fully educate their patients, put what's going on into non-specialists' terms, and be comfortable just skimming the surface. I could blame my lack of knowledge and many episodic flare-ups that caused my downhill exacerbations solely on the healthcare providers. It may be even easier to blame my parents had they not been invasive enough to have some continuous quest to find out the underlining factors of my prognosis. As I quoted are belated

Kobe Bryant, who believed failure wasn't an option, I was ready to submit to my failures. The only entity that was keeping my head above water what my grandmother and mother. Because of their two distinct love languages, their grit gave me the courage to muster my own.

Now, aware that my side effects never outweighed the benefits of these medications, I was reluctant to find others who also have experienced the same dead-end results. Although, if it means being the tail end of the stick, I can't support the negligence of big pharma and misguidance of doctors, as it's called in the United States, as a Trillion-dollar industry. These prescription drugs allow doctors to make millions. Yes, I agree some help maintain disorders and diseases but at what cost? How can we be more proactive in not facing taking these medications and their dire consequences? Doctors try to sell patients the drug because it's 'the newest and best drug on the market. Pharmaceuticals entice doctors with incentives to sell, and others prescribe the therapy while insurance and patents scrabble to keep up with costs. The pharmaceuticals are making killing. From two thousand to twenty eighteen, companies reported a cumulative revenue of eleven trillion and are skyrocketing. So are their cost. They said that "knowledge is power."

Spoon-feeding our children drugs further led to other ailments and chronicity. The medicines were disrupting my already fractured and fragile immune. The medications weakened my body's response to stimuli and made me defenseless. Practically, they are susceptible to infections that can lead to death, Immobility, compromised swallowing, respiratory disease, urinary tract infections, and cancers that may lead to the early demise of the patient. The decay of the nerve covering (myelin sheath) causes the complications associated with MS., Such as bacterial or viral infections that can make the immune system deficient and vulnerable. These complications are contingent on the fact that the immune system attacks itself. Our bodies attack our central nervous system as if it was foreign. Through proper diet, exercise, faith, a disciplined mindset, and creating healthier habits, rehabilitation of our immune system is most definitely possible, for I and many others have become a living testimony of this. Research, mindfulness, and support are some variables that helped change my circumstances, but I had to work through my pain. I had to forage almost fifteen years later of dare times until I stopped feeling sorry for myself.

Doctors opted only to tell my parents and me on a need-to-know basis, leaving many particulars out. They need to know what drug and how much it costs to be prescribed. They were left to read the pamphlets; unfortunately, they weren't interested in doing so, and neither was I. My mother entrusted the doctors with my life, but my grandmother didn't opt out of all other opinions, especially holistic ones. I felt obligated to take medication because I wanted to get better quickly. I was experiencing significant pain, and the lack of comfort was visceral. When I told the pains and symptoms I was experiencing, doctors, if I complained enough, they found no malice in playing Russian roulette with my health. My grandmother never left my health in the hands of doctors and western medicine. Manmie Lea was an old-school and phenomenal healer and elder.

Unknowingly, treatments were very costly - even twenty- three years ago, so when they found something, I was reluctant to take it, praying this would be the answer to all my problems. For years, I never considered how my mother paid for my medication and doctor visits; the most I understood was a co-pay. I never knew how the process worked.

My mother wanted the best treatment for me regardless of the cost. She was grateful that her job could give me the best insurance coverage. When that was over, how would I afford it?

Thus, as a black millennial child with MS, I was held hostage by the need to be cared for and dependent on medication. I figured I would never be able to care for myself. As I clung to my parents, my parents hung on to the doctor's every word. I was too young to understand, but I was desperate to alleviate my agony. I never had a choice of physicians, medication, or interventions. It was one thing after another. I was confused, angry, and resentful. Once diagnosed, the relief of knowing my diagnosis was very brief. It had no cure. What was I to do? I didn't just want alleviation; I needed treatment. I needed to dance again.

I had no choice but to go on whatever treatment I was prescribed, but at what cost? My back was against the wall, with pressure building in my mind and spirit. What was I to do but follow suit? My words turned to murmurs that were accepting accepted my prognosis. Because I couldn't come up with another option. I didn't know any better. I felt trapped and helpless. Doctors will claim it's the best drug but never mention its cost. It wasn't until Black American, groundbreaking television Emmy award-winning TV personality and comedian Richard Pryor was diagnosed with MS in 1986. Before then, he was known for his over-the-top comedic performances, which all racial audiences enjoyed. He poked fun at the division of white establishments and opened the conversation about racial division-wide. He was a drug abuser and attempted suicide by lighting himself on fire. The disease was even found in our narrative; doctors still did not think black people were afflicted. Richard Pryor lived out his life through the nineties in a wheelchair. He continued to perform with the chronic symptoms of MS. He became the first person to receive the Mark Wain Prize for American Humor from the Kennedy Center in 1998.

Died at sixty-five years old. Behold, this man didn't die of MS, yet he died of a heart attack. A year after my diagnosis, Montel Brian Anthony Williams, an American television host, actor, and speaker announced in 2000 that he was diagnosed with Multiple Sclerosis at nineteen- eighty-nine. He hosted his tabloid talk show, which ran from nineteen ninety-one to two thousand and eight. He served in the US Marine Corps and Navy for twenty-two years. Fantastic singer and songwriter Tamia, who has been former basketball player Grant Hill was diagnosed in 2003.

With recent populate, a rap feud began with rap artists Pusher T and Drake. Pusher T made a dis-record and targeted Drake through his best friend, Noah "40" Shebib. Pusher T raped about Ovo 40 illness. "... Hunch over like he eighty, tick, tick, tick" How much time he got? that man sick, sick, sick,' "40" was diagnosed in two thousand and five with MS. It was in poor taste, and Pusher felt the backlash. Amid the social media back last, "40" became an advocate with the National Multiple Sclerosis Society.

I was not familiar with these stories, coming from my community. I had never heard about Multiple Sclerosis in the black community, nor did I know anyone who had it personally. These names never resonated with me because I didn't see myself in their narrative. Besides Montel Williams, I had to research even to see a black woman with MS because of his social status.

By the time I caused wind of African Americans having MS, I wasn't the type of child to give care. Especially If it didn't grab my attention, my mind was all over the place, worrying about school, medications, doctor appointments, and playing to keep up with my normalcy. Their stories fell on deaf ears.

People don't die from MS. They die from all the disease complications and the side effects of the cocktail of medications. The infractions from all those things made me feel as if I was dying during my fight for survival. A war I was already told that I would never win.

This sort of dismemberment of the mind, body, and spirit seeps into my soul and corrosion my thoughts. One begins to feel a loss of purpose truly. Depression, anxiety, self-doubt, and lack of self-esteem took hold of me while I was in grievance because I had lost the child I once was.

Self-hate began to seep through the cellular walls and immerse itself in every cavity and crevice of my human anatomy. These symptoms started to surface and showed as fits, bursts of crying, laughter, or convulsions. The sudden loss of control of my bodily functions without explanation or origin made me emotionally unstable, severely sensitive, and depressed. My fatigue had me in a constant state of depression, falling asleep anywhere, in class at work, driving, during functions, meetings, in the middle of conversations, and everywhere else. One almost begins to adapt and succumb to the overwhelming feeling of helplessness and a mixture of hopelessness in all circumstances. This instability led me down a path of deep and dark depression. I have had trauma mentally, socially, and psychically and the inability to sustain productive and healthy friendships and moods. Depression is also a side effect of MS, and the medications I was given to treat MS. I became severely depressed throughout the years. Naturally, anything that changes the biological chemistry changes the flux of endorphins or lack thereof. I allowed statistical information to lead me rather than doing my research. The flesh is weak, but the young mind's naive loss of the normalcy I had before my diagnosis ultimately fueled my many lows because of depression and my view of the world around me.

Depression is the leading cause of suicide and suicidal attempts among patients with Multiple Sclerosis, with the stats being 50% more. I was affected and wanted to inflict as much bodily harm as possible. I wouldn't say I liked the weight gain from the steroids and the ineffective drugs the doctors continued to prescribe. I felt I was a liability to my family and all who encountered me.

My immune system went into system overload. My body would go haywire, or it would automatically shut down. I felt useless and began to feel shame. I resented myself because of everything I couldn't control. I could find the time to be happy anymore because I was too busy trying to be strong.

Some medications left my body available to contract any bacterial viruses and infections. I choose not to fight and give up and allow my body to succumb to the disabling circumstances; instead, my body folds under pressure instead of fighting against the disease, and the immune system crumbles. I had to combat Multiple Sclerosis with different therapies consciously, and I finally felt more alleviation.

On my most acute days, I was paralyzed or had double visions. In contrast, on other days, there may be numbness in the limbs, a tingling sensation, and twitching can also occur as hypersensitivity to heat and cold. I felt like a Raggedy Ann doll. On social media, I have met people from all walks of Earth, including and not limited to young women and men from Mexico to Indonesia and more. There's more substantial precedence in minorities than Caucasians. Multiple Sclerosis is also four times more common in women than men. Four hundred thousand people in America are steadily rising every year. In 2021 cases rose to two point one million worldwide.

Those who can neither empathize nor sympathize often take MS lightly. Since many of the symptoms aren't visible, people act as if they do not exist. The non-believers must look in-depth into one of the most widespread chronic neurological disabling diseases that is non-discriminatory.

Those who don't have the disease have a lack of understanding of the severity of the disease. I have been told to my face that I'm making it up because there are no apparent visual symptoms. It used to overwhelm me, but it no longer phases me as much because negativity toward the way I live no longer serves my growth. I work hard to sustain my new normalcy in Pediatric Onset Multiple Sclerosis, which accounts for one point two million patients under eighteen. I'm also more aware that I am no longer alone in my battles and that support begins and doesn't end with me. My story as a child ended but continues as a young adult. I was torn, poked, and supported by immense. This was the beginning of my plight and a lifetime of constant change. I'm two decades in, turning my pain and trauma into the guts and glory of my tomorrow.

No journey is real without resistance, hurt, and isolation, leading to an internal victory. After diagnosis, my life never got more manageable, it got more confusing, and I felt utterly alone but found my faith, vigilance, and pride to cast aside my doubts, and one day I'd be me again.

Welcome to My Tiny Spotted Mind